How to Fix Your Own Trigger Finger: The Journey Begins

Author
Ian Davidson PhD

ISBN 978-1-7395556-1-0

For Crixus and Xena
The "Poovaliers", Aaaah!

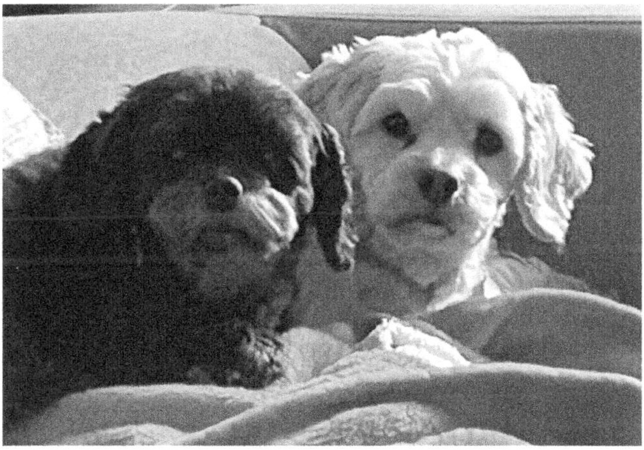

Little Rays of Sunshine

Illustrations by “*Schoolboy*”

"An investment in knowledge pays the best interest".

Benjamin Franklin 'The Way to Wealth' 1758

Table of Contents

Table of Figures

Note to Reader

This book is a self-help guide for people who have acquired trigger finger seeking treatment of a non-invasive nature and who have either received prior treatment that has failed or are looking for a naturalistic rather than a 'medical' or 'surgical' solution to trigger finger. All the treatments suggested in this book are based on simple remedies that have been referenced in other publications but not all have been tested as part of a randomised trial for the treatment of trigger finger. All have been clinically tested in various forms individually. This book presents temporally graduated, layered, combined interventions and a systematic method of measurement based on daily diaries and summary tables.

The treatments, approaches, mobilisations and massage techniques described herein are meant to supplement and not to replace or substitute for professional medical care or treatment. Diagnosis of trigger finger should be made by a competent health professional prior to engagement with the strategies in this book. The approach should only be applied after a healthcare professional has ruled out the possible other causes of symptoms that mimic trigger finger.

The treatments, approaches, mobilisations and massage techniques described herein are applicable only to acquired trigger finger in adults and NOT trigger finger (acquired, congenital or otherwise) in children. They are also not suitable for the treatment of trigger thumb which, because of its complex nature, requires a different approach. The treatments herein are only applicable to: digit 2 (index finger), digit 3 (middle finger), digit 4 (ring finger) and digit 5 (little finger).

People with the following conditions should not undertake any of the self-treatments presented in this book:

- Any vascular disorder including peripheral vascular disease or blood clotting disorders such as haemophilia.
- Have sensory deficits in the area being treated.
- Have an open wound (including burns or skin weeping as may be seen in psoriasis or other skin complaints such as eczema or impetigo, in the area that is being treated...).
- Unidentified and undiagnosed swelling or tumour in the area being treated.

- People who have been diagnosed with rheumatoid arthritis.
- Degraded or very thin, frail-looking skin.
- People with a diagnosis of amyloidosis.
- People with a diagnosis of mucopolysaccharidosis
- People with congenital trigger finger
- Children

In addition to these, there are some precautions, which are things that need to be considered as potentially adverse to the interventions made in this book. These are covered in more detail when considering the participants 'baseline' considerations in Chapter 1.

Preface

The British Association of Hand Surgeons in 2016 undertook an investigation[1] into the efficacy of treatments for trigger finger and concluded that although many treatments were available, they recommended that first line treatment should be a cortisone injection into the affected area and should this fail, surgery should be offered. This recommendation has been adopted by the National Institute for Health and Care Excellence (NICE) for management of the condition on the English National Health Service (NHS). On the face of it, this sounds all very reasonable except that an estimated 20% of the population are needle phobic[2] and many are reluctant to undergo surgery, partly through fear of adverse effects and partly because they are required to take time off work in the post-surgery period. This is particularly so for manual workers who may have to take several weeks off work after surgery.

To make matters worse, in 2018, the UK government restricted access to certain procedures which were considered "ineffective or risky" one of which was release of trigger finger[3] which is now considered a procedure of low clinical value (PoLCV)[4]. This means that surgery for trigger finger is now no longer a routine treatment but one which requires certain criteria to be met and for special dispensation to be made. This decision has seen the cost of surgery rise in the private sector from £600 per treatment to £3000 over a very short period of time.

This book is for ADULTS (not children) who find themselves with ACQUIRED TRIGGER FINGER (not congenital and not caused by a disease process) and are unable to find suitable treatments outside of the standard medical care offered. All of the treatments suggested in this book are established treatments which have been rejected as ineffective (but not risky) by a leading surgical think tank which has opted to recommend treatments that are medically orientated and within their sphere of knowledge and authority.

The methods outlined in this self-help book are readily available as "over the counter" solutions and have strong theoretical underpinning. Some provide estimates for success and are intended for less severe cases. This book also provides a series of outcome measurements collected in diary form to enable readers to monitor change over a prolonged period.

First of all, I would like to start off with a brief explanation: I am a UK neuro-physiotherapist and some years ago I acquired trigger finger. Naturally, because of the nature of my profession, trigger finger was, for me, something of a problem as my hands are central to my livelihood... as they are for many. To be honest, prior to acquiring trigger finger, I never really gave the condition much thought as it isn't something that would normally be treated by a physiotherapist. In my experience, and certainly in the books that you read about this and other hand conditions, it was felt that the best course of action was to have surgery to release the tissue.

To cut a long story short, I was able to find a way of dealing with trigger finger without using any medical interventions whatsoever. In other words, I did not go to a medical practitioner for a steroid injection and neither did I have surgery. However, I was able to successfully treat my trigger finger and following this, I developed a method of treatment for trigger finger that I call the ManTTr® Protocol about which I have written a separate book[5]. This current book that you are reading is not about the ManTTr® Protocol however, to some extent, it is a prequel to it. Let me explain:

The ManTTr® Protocol is a means by which trained therapists can intervene with patients to fix their trigger finger. It is not something that patients can apply to themselves. When I treated myself, I did so knowing that my case of trigger finger was quite mild and it was only on a "hunch" that made me intervened in the way that I did. At first, I wasn't even sure that the improvement in my trigger finger status was as a result of my intervention as it is estimated that between 20-30% of people spontaneously recover from trigger finger[6]. However, other indications suggested that this was not the case and it was on the basis of what I learned by treating my own trigger finger that I realised I could apply a more formal approach to effectively treat the trigger fingers of other people. This included cases that were more severe than mine.

Given that, in the ManTTr® Protocol, the treatment is offered by a third party, it would not be appropriate for me to describe it here as the book on the ManTTr® Protocol is written as a guide for therapists and as information and education for those who either have, or have an interest in, trigger finger. Much of the theory about why this type of intervention works is described in great detail in my book on the ManTTr® Protocol but now, I feel that there is an opportunity for me to explain to people who have trigger finger, particularly those with a mild form, how they may treat themselves. In the event that this self-help treatment does not work, there is always an opportunity for people to follow the ManTTr® Protocol as long as this is delivered by a component therapist possessing and appropriate skills. Should that fail, then there is no reason why the more invasive treatments of steroid injections and surgery could not be undertaken as a last resort.

In this book, I have therefore set out to bring together all of the standard treatments, no longer recommended by the UK medical profession for the treatment of trigger finger, not because they are dangerous or risky, but because they have been deemed to be ineffective. The reason that I am returning to these "traditional" approaches is because I do not feel that they have been given a fair airing as potential treatments either individually or in combination. I wanted to take a more measured approach by walking readers who have trigger finger through a series of interventions which, when replied consistently and progressively over a period of weeks, can bring about an improvement in the physical state of the trigger finger but also, and more importantly so that they might gain a deeper understanding of what is going wrong in the body that creates trigger finger. It is not possible to say whether this will work or not however, it is a means by which a person with trigger finger, particularly those who have a mild form, may take responsibility and charge of their own problem at minimal cost to them beyond the application of time and effort.

To that end, I present to you the book: "How to Fix Your Own Trigger Finger: The Journey Begins."

I.D. Stockport, Greater Manchester, UK 2023

Chapter 1: Trigger Finger: The Background

Trigger finger is also known as "trigger digit". It's posh Latin name is *stenosing tenosynovitis*. The reason it is called trigger digit is because it can include the thumb. However, the ManTTr® Protocol[5] was designed for trigger finger and not for trigger thumb, which requires a more complicated approach than that applied to trigger finger. So, although a common description of trigger finger is "trigger digits", we will describe it as trigger finger as the treatments outlined in this book only apply to the fingers, and not the thumb. Photo 1 clarifies the terms related to the digits on the human hand.

Photo 1: Various names of digits

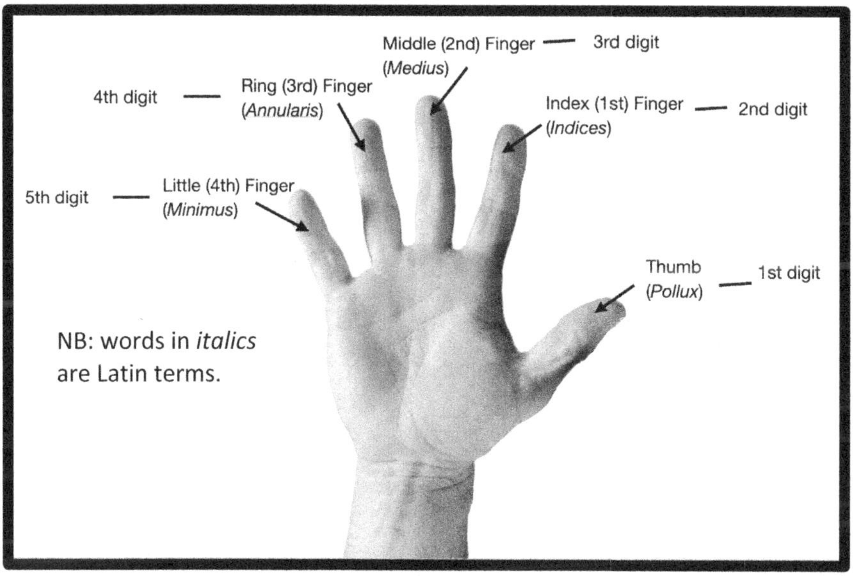

The mechanism of trigger finger

Although the cause of trigger finger is currently unknown, the mechanism by which the finger triggers during its archive movement is well documented. Typically, people with trigger finger experience a 'catch' or 'snap' when bending and straightening the digit[7] creating a 'roughening' of the movement in place of the smooth movement normally associated with the hand and finger.

Figure 1: Position of the formed nodule when the finger is bent

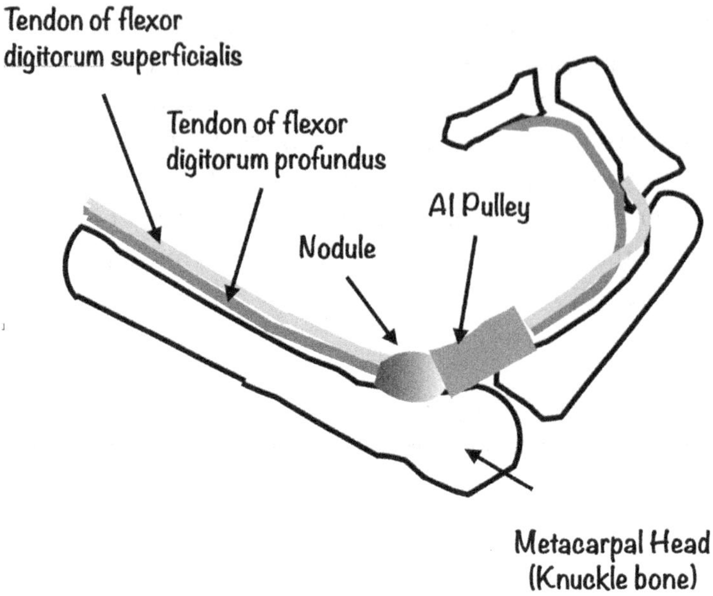

Figure 2: Position of the formed nodule when the finger is straight

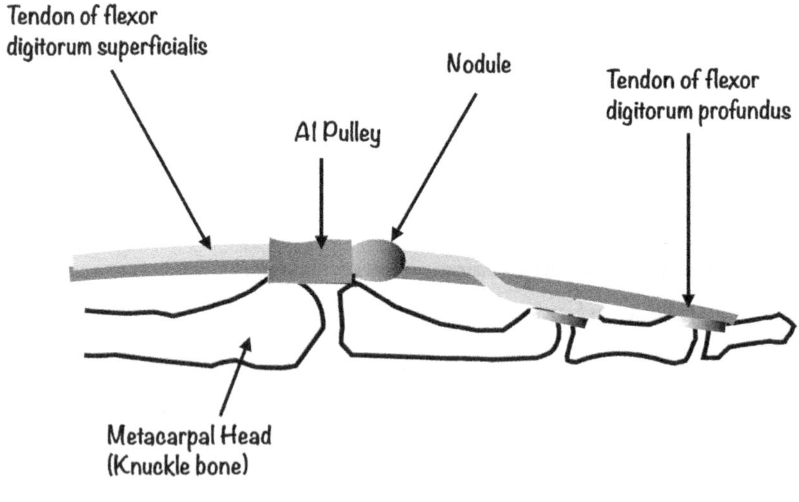

*Figures 1&2 adapted and reproduced with kind permission form the author and publisher of 'The Manual Therapy Trigger Finger (ManTTr®) Protocol[5]

This 'jerking' motion is created by a thickening of specific tendons as they pass in and out of a tunnel (referred to as the A1 pulley) located on the palm-side of the main finger knuckles which are known as the metacarpal heads[8]. Frequently, a painful lump in the palm, tender to pressure[8], is present. It is believed that this is caused by the development of a 'nodule' (soft tissue thickening) in the affected tendon. Figures 1 and 2 show the mechanism of this in relation to when the fingers are bent and when they are straight respectively.

The symptoms of trigger finger are most noticeable on waking when the hand is felt to be at its stiffest. Sometimes, people with trigger finger wake up with their hand squeezed tightly into a fist and find that when opening, the "clicking" of their digit is at its most severe and sometimes most painful. Frequently, it takes some time before the fingers loosen although, as the day progresses, the hand and finger activity increase[9] and sometimes, for a short period, the hand may even function normally.

Although spontaneous recovery can occur in around 20-30% of cases[6], the normal trajectory for trigger finger is one of general worsening. In the most severe cases, progression is normally caused by increasing pain, particularly when the finger "triggers". This can result in people with trigger finger avoiding movement and finding strategies to undertake activities which avoid the use of the affected hand. This, in general, makes matters worse, as the hand, when not moved through its full range of motion, can rapidly stiffen to the point where the finger is permanently bent and is immovable either under its own steam, or by the use of external force such as the opposite hand. Once things get this severe, the interventions recommended in this book will not work and neither will the more powerful ManTTr® Protocol[5]. The only solution is surgery. Bearing this in mind, we need to be clear about when self-treatment and third-party manual therapy can be effective. Generally speaking, self-treatment is best applied to less severe cases of trigger finger and the more severe ones (except for the most severe) by the application of the ManTTr® Protocol[5] by a skilled and competent third party. As such, we need to consider the various levels of trigger finger and in order to do that we need to measure severity in trigger finger.

Measuring severity of trigger finger

There are three key measurements that need to be undertaken to monitor progress (getting better), stasis (staying the same) or regression (getting worse) of trigger finger and these are: pain, quality of movement and function. Thankfully, there are two or three really easy ways of measuring the quality of movement and pain. I will come to these later but firstly, I want to say something about hand function.

Measuring function in trigger finger

This is an extremely complex issue because the human hand is unique in the animal kingdom. We have such a wide variety of activities that we can perform because of our incredible hand architecture and control mechanism. In many ways, our hands are the things which set us apart from our land-duelling mammalian cousins because variable prehension (all forms of grasping, seizing or holding performed by the hand) is so fundamentally important to human existence. This is essentially an artefact of our bipedal locomotor system, meaning that we move around on two legs rather than four. Our quadrupedal cousins on planet earth have four legs on which they walk and run whereas we only have two however, we all have four limbs. Our upper limbs provide us with the ability to manipulate objects and allow us to climb and crawl which is in common with many other species however we are the only species to write, play musical instruments, weave, manufacture... and do so many other things that cannot be done by other animals on planet earth.

So important are our upper limbs, that's our brain, which is also unique in the animal kingdom, allocates very much more computing power (neurons) to our upper limbs than it does our lower limbs. So, if we think about the architecture of the upper limb we can see that it has many joints such is the shoulder, elbow, forearm joints, the many joints that form the wrist and wrist complex, not to mention the joints in the hand itself. It also has a complicated arrangement of muscles that control these joints, and the whole point of the entire upper limb is to place the hand where it needs to be in order for us to interact with the world. If we think about the upper limb as having a series of pulleys and levers that form a structure akin to that of a crane which lies between the shoulder and the wrist, these are there merely to place the hand where it needs to go. So, when it comes to function, our hands are vitally important which means that problems in the hand can seriously impact on the way we interact with the world. This is why such supposedly trivial matters such as trigger finger are not at all trivial and should be treated with great seriousness.

Given that function is such a wide-ranging activity for the human species, and so varied when compared to other animals, it is often very difficult to measure. As such, we need to see function almost solely from a subjective point of view. By that, I mean that we need to decide, as individuals, what it is about our trigger finger that prevents us from interacting with the world in a way we desire. As such it is very difficult for me, within the context of this book and in the absence of a face-to-face discussion, to say to you what it is that impedes your function. This is something that you have to do. So, in order to facilitate this process, you need to do an exercise: In this exercise, you need to note all the things that bother you when you are trying to do something. For example, when I treat people who have trigger finger in my clinic, they might tell me that they have difficulty opening jars or that they find it difficult to drive or they have trouble using implements such as scissors or can openers and such like. The number of activities that are impeded as a result of the presence of trigger finger are numerous but may only be specific to you.

The reason I mention this at this juncture, is because an important element of this book is for you to monitor your trigger finger while at the same time perform different actions and treatments which, over a period of weeks and months will, for some, be effective in reducing the burden that trigger finger places on your life. To do this activity, you need to place this book aside and write down or record or think about all the activities that you would like to do that you can't do and/ or all those things that you find difficult to do and so avoid doing as a result of having trigger finger. You also need to record all those activities that you do which you find difficult but which you have no choice but to do, and which are impeded by your trigger finger. This list might be short or exhaustive, it doesn’t matter. Either way, once you've done this, pick the ONE which is the most irritating that is to say the ONE that you would most want to change. You need to note this problem down because this will be the key function that you will want to overcome and it is this function that you will measure success or failure of any intervention that you undertake in trying to reduce the impact of your trigger finger.

Measuring quality of movement in trigger finger

There are two common scales which measure the quality of movement in trigger finger. Often they are described as measurements of severity of trigger finger however, in my opinion , the severity of trigger finger is measured primarily as a combination of quality of movement, pain and impediments of function. If these three elements are combined, they give a far better picture of severity of trigger finger than merely one outcome measure.

You will see that these two quality of movement scales, known as the Quinnell Scale[10] and the Stages of Stenosing Tenosynovitis scale (SST scale)[11] the latter of which is sometimes called the Patel scale. The SST scale is really a refined version of the Quinnell scale. Both scales really only described the increasing level of catching or locking that takes place as trigger finger progresses. It does not take pain or function into account at all. Both scales can be seen below:

The Quinnell Scale

This was the original scale that measured 'movement grade' in trigger finger[10]:

0 Normal
1 Uneven movement
2 Actively correctable locking of the digit
3 passive correctable locking
4 Fixed deformity

The SST Scale

The Quinnell scale was later modified by Patel and Bassini[11] and called the Stages of Stenosing Tenosynovitis (SST) scale and is the preferred metric for use in clinical practice[8]:

1. Normal
2. Uneven
3. Triggering = clicking =catching
4. Locking of finger in flexion or extension unlocked by active finger movements
5. Locking of finger in flexion or extension unlocked by passive finger movement
6. Locked finger in flexion or extension

Measuring pain in trigger finger

Pain is generally measured in two ways. These are known as the pain numeric rating scale (PNRS) and the visual analogue scale (VAS). These are described below:

Pain Numeric Rating Scale (PNRS)

This is also known as the Numeric Rating Scale (NRS) and is commonly used by health professionals such as doctors, nurses, physiotherapists, psychologists, occupational therapists and others who are interested in the measurements of pain. An example of the PNRS is shown in Figure 3.

Figure 3:The Pain Numeric Scale

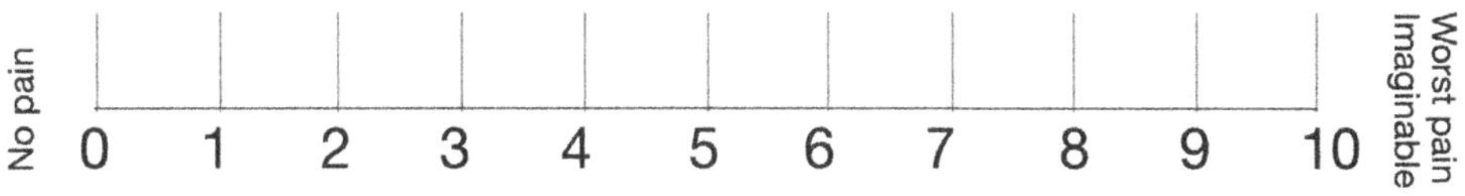

Essentially, it is a horizontal line which is marked off at equal intervals between 0-10, making this an 11-point ordinal scale. An ordinal scale, also known as a ranking or hierarchical scale, is one which has one interval higher or lower than the other but the interval is of an unknown quantity. In this scale, the zero towards the left-hand side in Figure 3 represents a point at which there is no pain whatsoever and on the opposite end, there is a point marked "10" which represents the worst pain imaginable[12]. If someone were to describe the pain that they are experiencing at any one time, for example, when assessing the pain experienced due to trigger finger, the person making the judgement would decide which of these numbers best represented the perceived level of pain. Of course, there is a downside to this: it is not possible to actually 'calculate' someone's pain and neither is it possible to compare actual pain levels between people however, it can tell you about pain **perception** for an individual at any given point in time and over a specific time period. Also, within a group of people, it can tell you if median perceived pain levels have changed following the application of specific interventions.

By that I mean, if someone on one day scores their pain at level 6 and then on another day they mark their pain as level 8 then this does not mean that their pain has gone up by 20%, but it does mean that their perception of pain has risen. Interestingly, this rise would not be considered important as the minimally important clinical difference (the MCID) is 30% on this scale[12]. However, if someone assesses the pain in their trigger finger as being level 8 when they wake from sleeping and level 2 in the middle of the day and then before they go to bed their pain is at level 5, then this tells us that the perception of pain fluctuates throughout a day. This is very valuable information to have if you have trigger finger and it is also very important information that you can give to a health professional if such a need arises.

The visual analogue scale

The visual analogue scale (Figure 4) is very similar to the PNRS in that it is a horizontal line and it has two extreme positions with the left-hand extreme being no pain at all and the far right being the worst pain imaginable[12]. Sometimes, there is a zero at the left-hand side and a "100" mark on the right-hand side. This is because the length of the line should be exactly 100 millimetres (10 centimetres) long.

Figure 4: The Visual Analogue Scale

Again, this scale measures perception of pain and again, is used widely throughout the health sector for people who have an interest in measuring pain perception. It differs from the PNRS because it does not have any markings on the line. In order for the person being assessed to give an assessment of their perception of pain, they would draw a mark on this line and the treating health worker would measure the distance from the left-hand side up to the mark on the line. This would be measured in millimetres. This is why this has a standard length of line, so that the measurement of pain would be out of 100. So, if somebody placed a mark in the middle of this line, then they would score 50. If after a period of time they reassessed their pain again, and they placed a mark on the line which was measured at 48, this would not mean that they had a 2% reduction in their pain and it is unlikely that this is a meaningful difference in perceived pain as it is very close to 50. However, if they were to mark the line at say 20 millimetres, then it could be presumed that there had been a general reduction in their perception of pain. This is because it is accepted on this scale that a change of 13.7 millimetres is considered to be the minimum size that is of clinical importance (MCID)[12]. Of course, the obvious downside to this scale is that it is difficult to see how pain can be measured in millimetres. However, that is to miss the point which is that this is not a measure of actual pain, but a measure of **perceived** pain whether or not this perception is rising, falling or staying the same. In that sense, it is used in exactly the same way as the PNRS. One advantage of the VAS over the PNRS is that it is difficult for someone to remember exactly where they placed the mark on the line, whereas it is very easy for a person to remember which score they gave on a previous occasion. However, if the they are responding faithfully, then this should not matter.

Self-Assessment

As with all interventions on the body, we need to have a baseline statement of our personal profile and current physical state of our trigger finger against which we are able to measure change. The programme set out in this book, requires you to undertaking some simple interventions to bring about change in your trigger finger and we need to measure the effect of these so you will need to establish a baseline.

We do this by completing a form that is pertinent to you and a full week of diaries recording your current state of trigger finger prior to undertaking any interventions. This is because trigger finger can vary day to day and so we need to get a picture of this variation.

In the section below, there is a database form for you to record details about you and your trigger finger. Don't worry, information will only be possessed by you because you are going to write it in your book! professional. It will give them a sufficiently detailed picture of your condition without having to go through a great many questions.

Table 1: Database for Trigger Finger

Database for Trigger Finger	
Date of Form Completion:	*Age (in whole years)*
Birth Gender (state... this matters!)	
How long have you had trigger finger in years and/or months?	
Dominant Hand:	☐ RIGHT ☐ LEFT ☐ BOTH (ambidextrous)
Fingers affected:	RIGHT Index☐ Middle☐ Ring☐ Little☐ Thumb ☐ LEFT Index☐ Middle☐ Ring☐ Little☐ Thumb ☐
Do you have any problems with the following: Heart: ☐ Lungs: ☐ Circulation/clotting disorder: ☐ Neuro: ☐ Conditions: e.g. Uncontrolled High Blood Pressure ☐ *State Specifics*:	
Do you have any of these conditions: Tick all those that apply: Rheumatoid Arthritis ☐ Type 1 Diabetes ☐ Type 2 Diabetes ☐ Amyloidosis ☐ De Quervain's Syndrome ☐ Carpal Tunnel Syndrome ☐ Hypothyroidism ☐ Gout ☐ Dupuytren's contracture ☐ Mucopolysaccharidosis ☐	
Occupation:	
Hobbies:	

However, should you decide or need, in the future, to seek 'face-to-face' professional help for this condition, the information recorded in this form, together with the daily diaries will be of great value to the attending health

For example, if you were seeing me, I would like to see this information (database and diary) prior to having a consultation as it would give me a clear picture of the background thus facilitating our consultation. It would also allow us to appraise the nature of your condition and allow us to determine whether it is improving, staying the same or getting worse. This is a very important aspect of the treatment of this and many other conditions. The initial database form can be seen in table 1. I will now explain why all of this information is necessary.

Significance of form information

The date of the form completion provides us with a 'time stamp' for the start of the intervention process. In a sense, it is a statement of 'taking action'! Once you have put at date on this form you must complete it straight away as a commitment to your journey beginning. Stating your age is important as it helps to 'profile' or 'place' you within the overall picture of people who get trigger finger. Typically, this is acquired in the 5th and 6th decades of life[9] which is to say between 40 and 59 (give or take) years of age. Just to clarify this point: when you are born, between the age of zero years to 9 years of age, you are in your first decade. When you turn 10, you enter your 2nd decade and when you turn 20 you enter your 3rd, and so on and so forth. This means that when you are 40 years of age, you have entered your 5th decade... scary, I know... at the time of writing, I have just entered my 7th decade!

Birth gender matters too, as females are 5 times more likely to acquire trigger finger compared to males[7]. The literature does not provide much of an explanation for this, but in my book on the ManTTr® Protocol[5], I provide a new theory for the development of trigger finger which gives a credible explanation of why females are more prone to trigger finger than males. This explanation is not covered in this book as this is not relevant to the purpose of this book which is merely to provide strategies to deal with trigger finger on a 'self-help' basis.

The length of time that you have had trigger finger is important as it gives us a sense of 'chronicity' both in terms of pain and tissue change[13]. Generally speaking, the longer you have had a condition, the more associated problems develop along with it. For example, the general trajectory of trigger finger is one of a worsening clinical picture as you get older as tissues tend to tighten naturally with age[14]. This is partly to do with the 'natural history' of the condition, in other words, that which is observed in the natural course of events and how our behaviour changes in response to the problem over time. Specifically, there is a tendency to adopt a strategy of 'hand-use avoidance' by finding ways round using our hand in certain 'painful' or 'awkward' situations. Essentially, it is a process of 'learned disuse'. This results in stiffening of affected and unaffected joint alike and this can make overcoming the problem of trigger finger more difficult.

Dominant side is relevant as the literature tells us that trigger finger is more common on the dominant side[8]. This is recorded on the database as it goes to 'your profile' or the extent to which you are 'typical' or 'atypical' of someone who gets trigger finger. Having trigger finger on your dominant hand can be most inconvenient but, surprisingly, it is probably a benefit. This is because it almost guarantees that the affected hand will be used and so hand use avoidance (or learned disuse) is less likely. Let's face it, it's much easier to avoid using your non-dominant hand than it is the dominant hand. If the non-dominant hand is affected, it is much more likely to deteriorate through disuse and so more complications are likely to develop more rapidly.

Related to this 'profile' issue, is the matter of which finger(s) are affected. The most common digit to be affected in people without concurrent disease is the thumb[6] but any finger can be affected. In general observation, the ring and middle fingers appear to be the most affected but multiple trigger finger is not uncommon and it can also be bilateral[7]. However, having multiple fingers affected on both hands is relatively rare. In terms of self-treatment, it might be better to treat the most problematic finger first to see if it brings about a change and then progress to the others. However, some might argue that the least affected finger should be treated first as this is likely to respond more quickly and with a more complete outcome. Others would argue that all affected fingers should be treated together. While this might be possible with the finger immersion technique shown later in this book, splinting might be problematic for obvious reasons.

The next section relates to your medical history and pre-existing conditions i.e. conditions you had prior to acquiring trigger finger or have recently acquired. These are listed so that you can review their present state in terms of their relative stability. Any condition that is unstable will require you to consult your physician before undertaking any additional treatment, including self-help treatments. As a general guide, if you require frequent visits to your doctor for medical reviews and tests then it is likely that there is a degree of instability about your condition. The main reason for requiring medical assurance relates to safety. It is not because the self-treatments offered in this book are aggressive or excessive, but some require immersion in heat and others the application of self-massage which could cause some discomfort.

For example, if you had labile (unstable) blood pressure (where your blood pressure suddenly rises and falls for no apparent or predictable reason) it would not be wise to immerse large areas of your body in warm water for extended periods. The reason for this is that when you are in warm water for extended periods, your blood vessels open and this reduces what is called the 'peripheral resistance' and this can lower your blood pressure which, in turn, can require your heart to beat more quickly. If this heart rate adjustment does not occur, the blood pressure may drop, causing a faint and this could be potentially dangerous. Another reason is that, with heart and lung problems, you may lack the stamina to undertake some of the activities that are required for the effective treatment of trigger finger. For these to have a chance of being successful, you need to be both **consistent**, that is, do the correct things, and **persistent**, meaning that you need to keep on doing them. Just picking at these interventions every now and again is likely to yield no positive results. As such, you need to ensure that you are fit enough to engage with the recommendations, as they require you to make daily interventions that are multiple in nature.

If you have a circulatory disorder, the blood flow to your tissues is compromised and so in terms of trigger finger, you will constantly be swimming against the tide as resolution of any inflammatory condition requires that the healing process is allowed to complete. If you have a circulation disorder, this completion of the healing cycle is often interrupted or never completed. Also, if you have a problem with clotting, that is, have a condition such as haemophilia or you are on drugs that make your blood thin, then you should not undertake the interventions recommended in this book. This is because you may experience very heavy bruising or, in the case of haemophilia, the very much more serious, haematoma which is caused by bleeding into the muscles. Under these circumstances, some of these interventions, particularly those relating to any kind of massage or mobilisation, are not recommended and even forbidden (contra-indicated). For example, you should not undertake these suggested interventions if you have amyloidosis, haemophilia, mucopolysaccharidosis or rheumatoid arthritis as these are systemic diseases that will not improve or will even respond badly to some of the physical interventions suggested in this book.

If you have neurological (neuro) problems, such as stroke, peripheral neuropathy, multiple sclerosis or any other condition, neuro or otherwise, that can impair your sensation, particularly relating to deep pressure and temperature, you should not perform these activities. For example, the application of massage or warm water immersion are not recommended as an inability to detect when water is too hot or when pressure is too great can result in damage to the tissues. It is recommended that in all conditions that you exercise caution and where you are uncertain, you should consult your doctor and/or other registered health professional for advice.

Pre-existing conditions must be well controlled and stable before engaging with the interventions recommended in this book. This could include something like high blood pressure or diabetes. This is because some techniques require the application of pressure over tissues and this might cause discomfort in some cases. Discomfort has been known to influence blood pressure and so caution should be heeded when applying these pressures. In the case of uncontrolled diabetes, even relatively minor tissue damage can result in suboptimal healing, possibly resulting in a worsening of the condition rather than the intended amelioration. However, the interventions in this book are considered relatively gentle and at no point is extreme heat or extreme pressure recommended.

The next section on the baseline data includes all known associated conditions with trigger finger: Rheumatoid Arthritis (RA); Diabetes (types 1 ad 2); Amyloidosis; De Quervain's Disease (Tenosynovitis) Gout; Carpal tunnel syndrome; Hypothyroidism; Dupuytren's contracture; and Mucopolysaccharidosis [11, 15, 16] are all related to an increased incidence of trigger finger. A brief overview of each condition is included in Table 2 below. Some of these conditions are known as 'systemic' conditions that precipitate trigger finger as part of a disease process. These include: Rheumatoid Arthritis (RA); Amyloidosis; and Mucopolysaccharidosis. These three conditions should not be treated using physical treatments for trigger finger because, in the case of amyloidosis, triggering is not caused by mechanical dysfunction but by protein deposits on the tendons themselves and these cannot be positively influenced by treatments of a physical nature.

In the case of rheumatoid arthritis, this is an auto-immune inflammatory disease of collagen (a ubiquitous protein in the body that connects everything to everything else) which is mediated through inflammatory processes and can, in some circumstances, deplete tissues to the point of creating spontaneous rupture of tendons and or ligaments. Furthermore, in inflammatory conditions, such as rheumatoid arthritis, the application of heat during exacerbations is not recommended as it is potentially deleterious to the inflammatory process.

In the case of mucopolysaccharidosis, this is a systemic condition that alters tissues in such a way that they are undermined, causing them to have systemic fragility, making them more prone to damage caused by pressure to tissues implicated in trigger finger. People with diabetes can undertake the interventions suggested in this book as long as the condition is in a consistent and medically stable state.

Table 2: Key Conditions Associated with Trigger Finger

Condition	Key relevant points about the condition [11, 15, 16]
Diabetes	A complex metabolic condition affecting the secretion/resistance to insulin production. Uncontrolled, it can create hyperglycaemia (too much sugar in the blood stream) causing structural degradation of soft tissues in humans[17] affected connective tissues, muscles, tendons and ligaments and is associated with sclerosis of tendon sheaths and collagen degradation[18]
Rheumatoid Arthritis (RA)	A systemic autoimmune pathology causing bouts of inflammation. Its autoimmune status means the body is unable to recognise certain proteins (collagen, histones, fibrin or fibronectin) as part of the body and so the immune system treats them as foreign bodies or antigens.[19]
Gout	A condition causing crystal deposits as a result of supersaturation of urate. It is an inflammatory arthritis characterised by painful attacks of joint pain. It is associated with metabolic syndrome, kidney disease and osteoarthritis[20].
Amyloidosis	The most common form is amyloid light chain amyloidosis, an ultra-rare, multi-systemic, incurable protein misfolding disorder. It undermines organ function resulting in multi-organ failure[21]. Another type of amyloidosis (wild type transthyretin amyloidosis) can be detected by the identification of amyloid deposits on the finger tendons which can cause trigger finger[22].
Hypo-thyroidism	A depletion of thyroxin production. Thyroxin is an important hormone in the metabolism, contraction, formation and repair regulation of skeletal muscle. Interruption of its production frequently causes muscle pain and fatigue[23]. Thyroid disfunction is common in people with metabolic syndrome (about 32%)[24, 25]
Carpal tunnel syndrome	The most common entrapment neuropathy of the upper limb causing compression on the median nerve precipitating pins and needles in the hand. Seen mostly in women aged 45-64 at a ratio of about 2:1 women to men. Idiopathic in origin, it has the following risk factors: High frequency, repetitive hand and wrist movements; obesity; pregnancy; osteo-arthritis of the MCP of the thumb; inflammatory joint disease e.g., RA causing synovitis in the carpal tunnel; Ganglion cysts, tumour, scar tissue; hypothyroidism; and diabetes mellitus. Management: conservative and then surgery[26]. Post-surgery, increased risk of trigger finger[27].
Dupuytren's contracture	A progressive fibro-proliferation disorder of the palmar fascia in the hand and fingers of unknown origin. Leads to disabling flexion contracture. It has higher prevalence in Northern Europe and is 6 time more common in men (peak mean age 55) compared to women (peak mean age 65). Other risk factors include: diabetes mellitus; smoking; high alcohol consumption; elevated serum lipids; hand trauma[28].
De Quervain's Disease (Tenosynovitis)	A degenerative stenosing inflammation of the tendon sheath of abductor pollicis longus (APL) and extensor pollicis brevis (EPB). Women represented 3:1 versus men. Peak incidence at the age of 40–59 years[29]. Risk factors: Diabetes, rheumatoid arthritis, lupus, and hypothyroidism[30].
Mucopoly-saccharidosis	An inherited metabolic disorder caused by a deficiency of specific enzymes that degrade important polysaccharides called glycosaminoglycans which can lead to damage to various tissues[31] including soft tissues, and particularly collagen[32].

*Reproduced with kind permission of the author and publisher of 'The Manual Therapy Trigger Finger (ManTTr®) Protocol[5]

Other conditions in this list such as: Gout; and Dupuytren's contracture probably precipitate trigger finger due to either acute or chronic biomechanical changes respectively. In the case of gout, if trigger finger forms during an exacerbation of the joint inflammation then self-treatments for trigger finger will not work. However, if the gout is dormant and trigger finger develops, there is no reason why the self-help protocols described in this book would not be appropriate. In the case of Dupuytren's contracture, particularly in moderate to severe cases, there is permanent severe fibrous tissue formation within the structures of the palm and so creates (in the absence of surgery) an immutable biomechanical abnormality where physical treatment for trigger finger would not be effective and so the protocols demonstrated and shown in this book should not be done as success is unlikely. However, this may not be the case in mild forms where Dupuytren's tissue has formed in the palm but there is no functional deficit and range of motion in the hand is unaffected. Under these latter circumstances, it might be worth attempting the interventions in this book.

Bearing these caveats in mind, the application of the protocols described in this book could be applicable in most cases. Possible additional exceptions are for people who have peripheral neuropathies or other neurological conditions where the sensation in the upper limb, and particularly the forearm and hand are impaired to the extent that they are unable to distinguish hot from cold, should not take part in the protocols and those with open wounds and serious skin irritations, rashes and skin diseases should not take part either. Also, given that some suggested self-treatment is given with the opposite hand, as a general point, people with dysfunction in the opposite hand would not be able to complete all of the suggested interventions and so these participants may not achieve the changes hoped for.

Finally, returning to our database, occupation and hobbies are important as frequently these require the hands to be used in particular ways. There has been suggestion that trigger finger can be caused by trauma to the hand particularly as a result of the use of hand tools[9]. Another reason for recording occupation and hobbies is because it reminds us of the things that we do with our hands during our work and also reminds us of the last time that we engaged in our hobby or if we avoid doing our hobby because of the problems we face with our trigger finger. Returning to a hobby could be one of our aims when considering the extent to which our function improves after an intervention, in other words, return to normal activity is a very good outcome measure.

Although the evidence for trauma to the hand or the use of hand tools is quite weak, it is interesting to note that despite the many millennia of medical practise, going back to the ancient Greeks and probably before, trigger finger was only first described in the late 19th century. To me, this speaks volumes about the nature of this condition in that it was identified at the height of the industrial revolution when factories were crammed full of people doing repetitive, monotonous, awkward, harsh work particularly with their hands.

The reason I find this interesting is because the situation found in these factories or "satanic mills" as they were once called, bring together all of the ingredients required to precipitate trigger finger. We don't need to go into the detail of this as the cause of trigger finger, as it is discussed and explained elsewhere[5]. What we can say though, is that the current living conditions that we have in the western world are still consistent with a mechanism that precipitates trigger finger to the extent that up to 3% of the population is likely to acquire it in their lifetime[7, 33]. For people with diabetes, it is estimated that at 10% of that population will get trigger finger[7, 33].

If you would like to see a video on the completion of the database for this book, please go to the following site:

https://www.youtube.com/watch?v=NVM3teeFaZs

The trigger finger diary

One of the most important activities that someone with trigger finger can do, is to monitor the progress or otherwise of their condition. In fact, I would go so far as to say that anybody with any condition would be well advised to monitor themselves. This is because, not only does it assist with communication with health professionals, but it also helps to understand what is going on and enables you to find relationships between activities that you are undertaking and the relative severity of the condition. For example, any condition that involves an inflammatory reaction (and most believe that trigger finger is one of these) then there is often a delayed response between performed actions and the symptoms that follow. This is because inflammation has a very strong temporal element, that is to say that it is related to time.

For example, migraine headache is associated with a range of potential precipitating factors. Although the universal cause of migraine headache is not known, there is growing evidence suggesting that many migraine caused by dysfunction in the cervical spine (the neck)[34-36]. However, despite this, certain "trigger factors" can precipitate migraine headache such as certain foods, certain visual stimuli and certain activities such as lying for too long, being overly active, being under active and so on and so forth. In attempting to find patterns to migraine headaches, it is advocated that migraineurs (people who get migraines) record daily headache diaries. In this way, they are able to identify patterns which are precursors, that is, factors that precipitate not only the frequency, but also the duration and intensity of migraine attacks.

The use of specific diaries to track symptoms and progress within a particular condition in healthcare is very common. Some conditions that benefit from the use of diaries or 'symptom journals' include: asthma, diabetes, eating disorders, multiple sclerosis, psoriasis, inflammatory bowel disease and even to assess the effectiveness and or side effects of medications. Each of these will have specific reasons for recording certain things but for trigger finger, the key data to collect are:

- Quality of movement and pain at three time points in the day (on awakening; during the most active part of the day; and prior to going to bed).
- Record sleep disturbance
- Comments about the functional status of your trigger finger in day.
- Record medication, frequency and dose for the condition each day.
- Fist formation and hand straightening.

The outcome measures chosen for quality of movement and pain are the SST (in modified form) and the PNRS respectively. Although others have been considered, I have decided to recommend these two because they are simple to use and understand, quick to make a note of as they are numeric and provide sufficient detail about the trigger finger to assess severity. However, as indicated above, I have slightly changed the SST to a more understandable form whereby 'normal' is ranked as zero and I've also changed the wording so that it is personalised to you. However, the overall description of the scale that is used within the diary, is very close to that of the SST scale[11]. So let us now take a look at the diary that you will be completing each day for the next several weeks and months.

As you can see in Table 3, the version of the calendar that I have used relates to **Week 0, Day 1**. So, let's take a look at the diary: Firstly, at the top left, we put the date that we are filling in the diary. This is to make sure that when you come to review and summarise your diaries at the end of this self-treatment process, you will see that you have been taking recordings on consecutive days. Continuous recording is important as it allows us to plot change more accurately on summary charts at the end of the series of interventions that you will perform... more about those soon. In this next section, we are going to record pain and a *modified* SST score at *three different time points in the day*. The 'key' for the pain and modified SST scores is written on the next two sections which are entitled **"Modified SST (stages of stenosing tenosynovitis) Score Key"** and the **"Pain numeric rating scale (PNRS) key"**.

NOTE: IF A BOX IS 'GREYED OUT' IN THE DIARY, IT SHOULD NOT BE FILLED OUT.

You will notice that I have used terms like '...waking after main sleep' rather than 'waking in the morning' as not everybody sleeps at night. Night workers, for example, sleep during the day and this will be their most important period to measure because it is at this point that their trigger finger is most likely to be at its stiffest, and possibly, most painful. As such, this is our most important measurement.

If, on Table 3, we go down in rows, the next measurement relates to the "most active period" of the day. This is usually the midpoint of our waking hours and normally, our best period of the day for trigger finger symptoms. In less severe cases of trigger finger, symptoms can disappear altogether. In more severe cases, say grades 3 and 4 on the modified SST scale (4 and 5 on the SST proper) pain levels may be less, but the quality of movement is likely to remain poor. On the next row is the modified SST score just prior to our main sleep. At this point, the hand will feel as though it is stiffening up and the pain levels may be rising.

Table 3: Example Daily Diary

Trigger Finger Daily Diary		Week 0	Day 1
Date:		**Modified SST score (see Key) 0-5**	**Pain Level (PNRS) (see key) 0-10**
On waking after main sleep	At rest		
	On bending/straightening		
During most active period	At rest		
	On bending/straightening		
Just prior to main sleep	At rest		
	On bending/straightening		

Modified SST (stages of stenosing tenosynovitis) Score Key:
0 Normal finger movement
1 Uneven finger movement (looks smooth but feels rough)
2 Triggering or clicking or catching (looks a bit jerky, not fully smooth)
3 Finger locking in a bent or straight position but can unlock by active finger movements
4 Finger locking in a bent or straight position but unlocked by passive finger movements
5 Locked finger in bent or straightened position but cannot be unlocked at all

Pain Numeric Rating Scale (PNRS) Key												
No pain	0	1	2	3	4	5	6	7	8	9	10	Worst pain Imaginable

My trigger finger today has:	**Yes**	**No**
Disturbed my sleep		
Prevented me from doing an activity I wanted or needed to do		
STATE AND DESCRIBE ACTIVITY:		

Medication for Trigger Finger: Frequency....................times/day **Medication Name: Total daily dose:**	**Yes**	**No**
Can you make a full fist just before my main sleep?		
Can you straighten your fingers fully just before my main sleep?		

If interventions are being effective, the one that we are most interested in, is the one on waking after the main sleep. If you notice that there is a change in this figure, then this often heralds future improvement in the trigger finger. However, you must continue recording the other two as there is often a slight delay in these and we need to calculate the rate of change in terms of how many days does it take from an improvement on waking after the main sleep, to recording improvement at the other two time periods. If we begin to see these changes, this bodes very well for trigger finger recovery.

The next part we need to complete, in our daily diary, is that section entitled "my trigger finger today has:" and then there are 2 things that we need to report on. The first of these is about disturbed sleep. Sometimes it's difficult to know whether you were woken up because of pain caused by your trigger finger or for some other reason. Let's face it, waking up in the middle of the night is not uncommon for many people.

As such, you need to make a judgement as to whether painful trigger finger was the primary reason why you woke up. Normally, as a rule of thumb (excuse the pun) it would not be unreasonable to say that it had woken you up if, when you awaken in the middle of the night, your hand is hurting. If you wake up in the middle of the night and your hand is not hurting, then the reason why you woke up is unlikely to relate to your trigger finger. Of course, this is overly simplistic, but at least it is, kind of, standardised. So, in this way, we can monitor the extent to which the trigger finger causes pain at night whether or not the reason for waking was truly the trigger finger. Also, for some, the problem is that the pain in the trigger finger is the cause of not getting to sleep in the first place. If this is so, and you are convinced that the trigger finger pain is the cause, then record this as 'your trigger finger is disturbing your sleep' in the diary. If the treatment is successful, this pre-sleep problem should abate.

The next row refers to reduced ability to do something that you wanted or needed to do. This could be anything to do with your work or hobby or interest or activities around the house or in the garden. It only has to be something that you wanted to do, were asked to do, needed to do or was merely intending to do. This has to be to do with your trigger finger however, it could have been a marginal activity by which I mean, it was something that you may have been able to do but decided not to do just in case you aggravated your trigger finger.

Therefore, this section is a measurement of the degree to which your trigger finger interferes with your life. This is something that probably happens to you all the time, possibly more frequently than you think, but which only now you will record formally and by doing this, you will be able to count how many days in any 7, that your trigger finger interrupted a functional component of your life. Highlighting this is important as it will make you take action to improve the state of your trigger finger and it will make you realise how much hand avoidance activity you are engaging in. This too is important as the avoidance of using your hand predisposes (makes more likely) to progression in trigger finger and complications in the hand such as weakness and stiffness.

The next part of the diary relates to medication that you take for trigger finger. There are three things that you need to record here: firstly, the frequency of how many times in the day have you taken medication for your trigger finger. The second is the name of the medication or its purpose, that is, whether it is an anti-inflammatory or painkilling medication. If you are unsure, put the name of the medication into one of the on-line National Formularies and it will tell you what the indications are for the medication, the side effects, interactions among other things. The British National Formulary (BNF) is a very good one and is free to use. It can be found via the National Institute for Health and Care Excellence here: https://bnf.nice.org.uk. Just type the medication name in the search bar right at the top of the page in their website. If you would like to see a demonstration of a search of the BNF, take a look at this video link:

https://www.youtube.com/watch?v=OrE8tDlgvdU

Finally, the total daily dose needs to be entered in your daily diary. So, for example, if you were taking 500 milligrams(mg) of paracetamol three times a day, that means that your total daily dose would be 1500mg. Recording medication use for a specific purpose is extremely important as it is an excellent proxy marker for the need for pain relief. The fewer medications that are used, generally indicates a lower level of severity. However, having said that, many people these days shy away from using medications as they feel that they add toxicity to their bodies. I have to admit, I am one of those people and will only take medication if I absolutely have to.

Finally, the diary ends by asking you if you are able to make a full fist before you settle down for your main sleep and whether or not you were able to straighten your fingers fully before your main sleep. The reason that this is asked at this juncture, is that these activities measure whether or not your hand has re-established its full range of motion. Being able to make a full fist or being able to fully straighten your hand and fingers before you go to sleep is a good sign as it shows that the pliability of the tissues in your hand are at their maximum mobility after having been used throughout the day. It will also allow you to have an appreciation of the degree to which your hand stiffens overnight. This is usually a marker of the presence of inflammation. If you are able to make a fist before you go to sleep and you wake up and your hand is stiff and you are unable to make the same fist, this shows that the tissues in your hand have tried to bind together overnight and this is a characteristic of an inflammatory process taking place.

You can see a video of me demonstrating what constitutes a full fist and a straightened hand and fingers, in the following link:

https://www.youtube.com/watch?v=pM-dCsK-XKM

If you would like to see a video of me filling out a fictitious diary, please go to the following link:

https://www.youtube.com/watch?v=lCbrU1Nxsq8

In the following chapter, I want to tell you how to use this book. As its title suggests, it is a self-help book for the treatment of trigger finger using basic methods of treatment that I walk you through step-by-step, in a systematic manner, to enable you to progressively explore and learn about how your trigger finger responds to these various treatments. This will take some work on your part and this work might have to go on for a number of weeks and possibly even months. However, it will cost you practically nothing except for some time and possibly some very minor equipment although this latter element may not be necessary as homemade alternatives are available.

Central to the success of this approach, is the requirements for you to record your journey in a series of diary entries. These diaries take only a few minutes to complete and are all set out for you below. All you have to do is complete the diary each day in the way previously described in this book and via a video link. You can do this from the next time you wake up. You need to complete a diary on consecutive days and while you are completing this diary over this week I will give you information about what is to come in the week ahead so that you can plan ahead.

However, it is important that you do not "jump the gun" and do things prematurely as you must do the things that I suggest in the order that I suggest them. The reason for this is that success or failure (and as failure, I would include 'stasis' that is to say that there is no change even though the natural history of trigger finger is to get worse) gives us information about how your trigger finger is responding and what is causing and perpetuating your trigger finger symptoms. It is possible that, while on this journey, you may need to add more of one thing and reduce other things and that this might be done at different time intervals. I know this all sounds a bit cryptic but as you read through this book, you will see that there is logic applied at every stage. So, don't delay the recording of your diary entries, this can happen as of the next time that you wake up from your main sleep. You don't have to wait for Sunday or Monday because we take the 7-day cycle from wherever it begins! With that said, let's now move on how you might specifically use this book.

Chapter 2: Week 0: Baseline and Daily Diary.

The first thing you need to do, which you can do right now, is to complete the database form, which gives your background and current relevant state. This is important because by doing this, you are becoming physically engaged in the process of improving your condition. The next thing that you can do, when you wake up from your main sleep, whenever that may be, is to begin completing the diary for Week 0, day 1 and everyday thereafter. The third thing I want you to do is to look at your palm and straighten your fingers.

On your finger that is triggering, I want you to place the thumb of your opposite hand over the most painful part of your hand. Do this gently and without significant pressure. If you have trigger finger, you will almost certainly feel a raised area underneath the most painful point in the finger which will probably be the part of the palm closest to the finger that is triggering. If you don't have any pain, feel around for a lump and then close and open your fingers and you will feel this lumpy tissue move. Now place your index finger of your other hand over the back of your triggering hand, placing it opposite your thumb of your opposite hand. Now gently roll your thumb around the raised area but do not apply any meaningful pressure. All you are doing here, is merely identifying the raised area which, in most cases, is a nodule, or thickened area, that is responsible for the triggering (Photo 2).

I want you to enjoy this moment because this is the last time that I want you to do this. I will come to why I don't want you to do this shortly but in my experience of treating trigger finger in my clinic, nearly everyone that I have treated has told me that they have been told to massage this area believing that it will "soften" or "break down" the tissue to free it and that this may ease the situation or even resolve the problem. Experience suggests that this is not so and in fact, in most cases, it creates irritation and perpetuation of the problem. So now that you've had a prod about in this area, you can now stop it forever because, in my opinion, it has no place in the treatment of trigger finger.

The next thing I want you to do is again, hold your palm in front of you and put the tip your index finger of your opposite hand on the fingertip of the finger that is triggering. I then want you to apply gentle pressure over the fingertip of your affected finger and bend it slightly backwards. After a couple of seconds note how this feels and then release the pressure. Now I hope you enjoyed that action too because it is the last time that I want you to do it until further notice. Doing this exercise is a hit and miss action, that is to say, sometimes it will be effective and sometimes it will not. Again, I will explain shortly why this is the case but for now, if you have been advised to do this (and I know that many people will have been) I would like you to stop it!

Photo 2: Nodule Massage

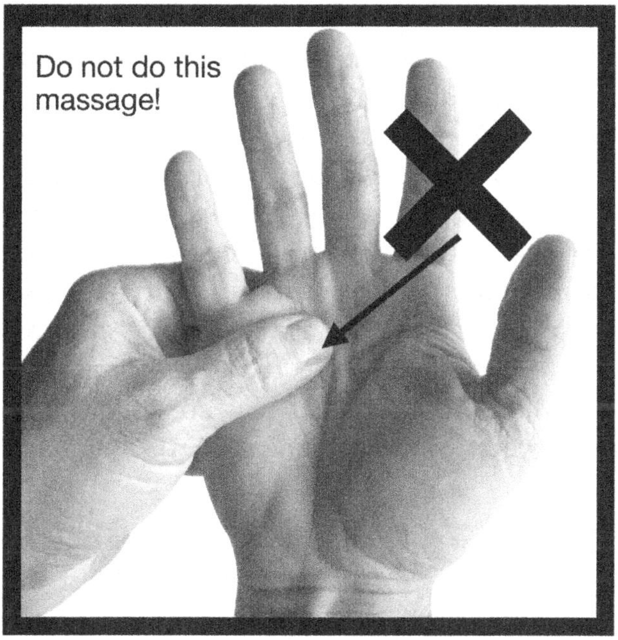

So far, I have given you three things to do right now and one thing to do when you next wake. The first thing is to complete the database and the latter 2 things that I wanted you to do is to stop doing them if you are doing them. The reason I've included these last two things that I **don't** want you to do, is because I know that these are commonly recommended when you search on the Internet. Now it is true to say that some people, having done these things, will have experienced a resolution of the trigger finger, but it is unlikely to be anything to do with these two particular actions and it is highly likely that their trigger finger would have resolved anyway, as is observed in up to nearly 30% of cases[6]. You will notice that, when these things are advised, those advising give very little underlying theory as to why the suggested approach might work beyond saying that it causes a "lengthening of the tissues" or it produces "softening of the tissues" or it "mobilises the tissues" which are explanations that are weak and unfounded. Some might say, for example that massage 'breaks down' the scar tissue which is, in my opinion, clear nonsense (see Photo 2). Scar tissue is fibrous tissue and is incredibly tough. WARNING- THE REST OF THIS PARAGRAPH IS ABOUT EATING MEAT... VEGANS AND VEGITARIANS MAY WANT TO SKIP THIS BIT: For the meat eaters out there, I'm sure that you have, in the past, bitten into some meat and found a piece almost impossible to break down with your molars. More often than not, the chewer removes the 'gristle' from their mouth as no amount of chewing can break the tissue down despite the molars of the average male being able to exert a force often in excess of 150 pounds per square inch (psi) and the average woman 110psi. As such, it's highly unlikely that massaging by use of your thumb is going to 'break down' this type of tissue. What's more is that the 'meat gristle' is dead and so weaker than live tissue which has better resilience. There may be some effect from the massage but this is more to do with the tissue repair cascade than breaking anything down. My recommendation therefore is to cease and desist from doing this throughout the whole of the period you are following my suggested method of treating your own trigger finger. NOTE- IT IS MEAT FREE FROM HERE:

Okay, so let's consider these interventions for a moment and think about what they do. But before we do that, we need to just think about the prevailing view of what is happening at the point of the nodule formation in the palm. Let's start with the posh name for trigger finger, which is 'Stenosing Tenosynovitis'[8, 9], and what this means: 'Stenosis' means narrowing and this relates to narrowing of the tunnel through which the tendons pass. 'Teno' means tendon, 'syno' means the synovial sheath that covers the tendon and 'itis' means inflammation. So, to translate, Stenosing Tenosynovitis means: inflammation of the synovial sheath and the tendon which passes through a narrowed opening. The minimum that we can glean from this is that it is believed that inflammation at the point of the thickening is an active contributor to the signs and symptoms of trigger finger[8, 9]. To reinforce this view, it should be noted that the accepted first line treatment for trigger finger in most developed countries is a cortico-steroid injection which has the putative aim of reducing swelling in the area presumably caused by swelling[6]. Cortico-steroids are one of the most potent anti-inflammatory drugs used by healthcare professionals and it should also be added that the success rate of this treatment is estimated to be around 60%[11, 37]. However, these estimates are based on a follow-up period of no longer than four months[6] and so the long-term effect of this treatment is currently uncertain.

So, if inflammation is a key ingredient producing the signs and symptoms of trigger finger, what effect do you think massaging over an inflamed area might have on those tissues, particularly if those tissues are in an enclosed space? Those of you who think that it would exacerbate the inflammation, you are likely to be right. This is why many people report that massaging the nodule actually increases the pain at the site of the triggering and yet they continue to do it in the belief that it is doing some good holding with an attitude of "no pain, no gain!" Now, don't get me wrong, this particular saying has some credence in some respects put massaging or manipulating over an inflamed area does not make sense! If you had an inflamed knee or ankle, would you advocate doing a deep massage over this tissue? I doubt it! There is no doubt that as the inflammation becomes more chronic and less active, there may be a case for some kind of soft tissue mobilisation but where there is acute inflammation, which may or may not be so in trigger finger, the case for deep soft tissue mobilisation becomes weak.

So now let's consider the issue of stretching the finger backwards which is intended to be a stretch (often called a tendon glide or elongation) of the affected tendons. Now, I must admit that I do sometimes used this, but my objection to its universal use relates to the unthinking nature by which it is recommended. As we go through this book, we will return to this exercise but we will do so with some thought rather than using it as a "scattergun" approach to its application. There is no doubt that it could be beneficial under certain circumstances however under others, it will make the signs and symptoms worse. I explain this in detail in my book "Manual Therapy Trigger Finger (ManTTr®) Protocol[5], but even if we think about this at a superficial level, we see that when we stretch the finger backwards in the way that I described earlier, we are stretching multiple tissues. These include the tendons which control the small joints in the fingers, the ligaments over the front of the joints beyond the palm, the synovial sheath covering the tendons, 3 fibrous pullies located in the finger and 2 strong muscles located in the forearm that control the tendons that bend (flex) the fingers.

Given that we know that trigger finger is a condition which grinds on for a long time, and we know that people who have trigger finger also lose range of motion as a result of hand use avoidance strategies (which Is also known as 'learned disuse') any one or combination of these tissues being stretched could be irritated. It is also possible that the tendons that are inflamed around the nodule would be irritated by a sustained stretch along their length, causing more irritation and possibly inflammation. On the other hand (excuse the pun) a stretch of this type could lengthen and free tissues from one another and so bring about a benefit. The point is, that at the time of making the stretch on the finger, we don't know what is actually happening. As such, this stretch, and similar stretches, must be done in a graded and specific manner and must not be used as a "scattergun" approach to lengthening tissues either related or peripheral to triggering finger.

So now that I have explained to you the reason why I do not want you to do these activities, I hope that you will refrain from doing them even though you may have been told to do them by via some other source. Of course, you can ignore my advice if you wish, but in doing so, you may well have wasted your money on buying this book. However, given that you have paid your solid legal tender for this book, it would make sense that you would at least give my advice the benefit of the doubt and follow my suggestions to the letter as we walk through the various things that I both want you to do and do not want you to do. You can judge for yourself by the end of the book as to whether you think my advice is sound or not. In fact, I would love to hear from you if you have any comments, and if you do, you can e-mail me at the e-mail address given at the back of this book. If you do contact me, please make sure that in the subject heading you put: "trigger finger self-help". Thanks!

So now we come to something which is quite controversial and that is the thorny question of using anti-inflammatory medication which can be bought over the counter without a medical prescription. I think this is such an important element of what I have to say, that I want to give it its own subtitle:

To anti-inflammatory or not to anti-inflammatory?

Non-steroidal anti-inflammatory drugs (NSAIDs) are the single most used medications in the world with between 5 and 10% of all medications used falling into this category[38]. They are easily available as over the counter medications and are inexpensive. There is no doubt that the literature tells us that the use of anti-inflammatory agents, which can be taken orally, given as an injection or applied topically (on the skin) in the form of creams or gels, are indicated in the treatment of trigger finger[39]. The most powerful of these are those which are injected directly at the point of pain in the hand. These have been seen as a possible alternative to cortico-steroid injections which are contraindicated (mustn't be used) for diabetics who have poorly controlled blood sugar, those with infections or those who are immuno-suppressed[39].

However, in my opinion, there is very little benefit in using anti-Inflammatory drugs in any form for trigger finger. Now that might seem to be an odd statement given that I have already intimated that an inflammatory process may be at the heart of the problem with trigger finger which is centred at the point where a tendon enters a tunnel called the A1 pulley. Well, here are my reasons: First of all, if NSAIDs are used, the most powerful means by which it can be applied is via injection directly to the point of pain in the hand. However, to do this, there needs to be a registered practitioner involved. This means that this approach no longer is an 'over the counter' treatment and so, given that a steroid injection is considered marginally superior to NSAIDs[39], cortico-steroid injection would be the preferred treatment. Moreover, while NSAIDs can be used for diabetics with poorly maintained blood sugar, the provision of treatments under these circumstances invites a degree of moral hazard in that there is a disincentive for diabetics to take control of their blood sugar which is essential to prevent further deterioration of body systems. However, the case for the use of NSAID injections for those who are immunosuppressed (bearing in mind the immunosuppressive effects of steroid injections)[40] remains.

The most likely means by which people take anti-inflammatory medication is through over the counter medication in tablet form. This is used widely for the treatment of musculo-skeletal disorders[41]. Oral medications (and to some extent topical agents) have a systemic effect on the body because their use allows the active agent to enter the bloodstream. However, regardless of the method of delivery, another argument against the use of anti-inflammatory agents, in any form, is that inflammation is an important stage in the body's natural response to healing, which is called the 'wound healing cascade' and as such, it could be argued that its artificial interruption is potentially harmful to soft tissue healing[42] and even, bone fractures[43]. Furthermore, in the case of oral anti-inflammatory agents, there are also potential side effects such as gastrointestinal, cardiovascular and kidney problems[38, 44] among others particularly with long-term usage[41, 45]. Added to this, from an anecdotal point of view and from experience of treating people who have trigger finger, this sort of medication taken orally or topically does not appear to be very effective. As such, viewing this in the round, it could be argued, that on a risk-benefit assessment, that the use of anti-inflammatory medication for trigger finger should not be advised.

On a final consideration on this matter, parts of the literature on trigger finger have suggested that it may not necessarily be an inflammatory disorder as histological studies, have no inflammatory cells present around the affected tendon[6] and that any inflammatory cells tend to be localised only to the synovial sheath covering the tendon[9]. The explanation may lie in the observation that tissue affected is swollen and tender with peritendinous fibrosis[46], meaning that the outside of the damaged tissue is thickened (but not inflamed) and sensitive to pressure.

Here lies a conundrum: firstly, if this is not an inflammatory condition, then why do corticosteroids appear to work in about 60% of cases and secondly, why does the fibrous nodule form, causing the tendon to become stuck in the tunnel? Well, in answer to the first question regarding the use of cortico-steroid injections, it is possible that the action of this drug under these circumstances is not anti-inflammatory but mechanical. That is to say that the insertion of fluid at a point where the tendon passes through its sheath where a nodule has formed, may be enough to change the fluid dynamics in the area in such a way as to create a biomechanical change in the area and thus ameliorate the problem. This, of course is conjecture however it seems rather suspicious that's the outcome for NSAIDs, given as an injection, have a similar outcome to cortico-steroids. The slight domination of cortico-steroid injections over NSAID injections is possibly due to the fact that the former is normally delivered together with a pain killing injection thus giving it a slightly longer duration of effect.

There is also the possibility that both are very powerful placebos given that we know that the placebo effect of injections can account for as much as 78% of change in back pain[47] and observably high rates in migraine headach[48, 49]. Finally, the success of steroid injections (or NSAID drugs for that matter) may depend on whether or not the root cause of trigger finger has an inflammatory components or not. In cases where inflammation is indicated, such as that described in the literature as inflammation of the synovial sheath covering the tendon, anti-inflammatory agents are likely to be effective. If inflammation is absent, then they are unlikely to be effective. This whole question turns, therefore on whether or not inflammation exists. It would be useful therefore if we could adopt strategies that gave an indication as to whether or not inflammation was the cause of the pain or if there was some other mechanism. We will discuss this a little later in this section.

Returning to the second question regarding nodule development; this is less easy to explain other than to opine that this is something which develops over a long time, possibly in relation to frequent irritation of the tendon possibly caused by faulty biomechanics[27, 50]. Once the nodule has reached a critical size, and is unable to pass cleanly through the tunnel created by the A1 pulley, when the fingers are bent and straightened, the nodule enters the tunnel formed by the A1 pulley and in doing so, compresses the synovial sheath creating inflammation on the sheath's inner surface. The formation of the nodule therefore could be as a result of repeated traumas to the same part of the tendon, thus creating minor, sub-symptomatic inflammatory reactions which go unnoticed. However, frequently repeated events eventually 'grow' the nodule in a progressive series of 'onion rings', with each inflammatory layer resolving and finally aggregate into a fibrotic thickening.

These explanations are plausible yet unproven. Either way, the argument presented here for the avoidance of anti-inflammatory medication is made. However, there will be readers who believe that anti-inflammatory medication, with or without pain killers, has a beneficial effect. To those people I would say this:

1. it is your body and, presuming you are a sane adult, you may do with it as you wish.
2. Always read the label of any medication you take and heed warnings and advice.

3. Always consult a registered medical or pharmaceutical practitioner before taking NSAIDs particularly if you have a known chronic condition or take other medication.

Finally, I would suggest that the solution to trigger finger does not lie with anti-inflammatory treatments (or painkillers) but in interventions related to tissue pliability and biomechanical realignment. A detailed account of how this occurs is documented in my book on the ManTTr® Protocol[5] but "ManTTr®" is not designed as a self-help guide, but a guide for therapists and bodyworkers. However, it is written in a style suitable for those who have trigger finger as a source of educational interest. In my opinion, for trigger finger, anti-inflammatory medications are merely palliative (symptom suppressing). Part of that palliative effect is to diminish pain, making the discomfort more manageable, as NSAIDs have both analgesic and anti-inflammatory effect[43]. Painkilling medication is a double-edged sword in that, in one respect, it relieves pain and allows the continuance of function and in another, it perpetuates soft tissue damage caused by strain on dysfunctional tissues.

So now that we have considered some things that we should, in my opinion, not do, we now need to consider those things that we need to do. However, I do not want you to do this until you have **completed** the Week 0 of your diary regimen. So, bearing in mind that it will take you seven days to complete your first week of diaries, you might want to think about planning for your first week of specific treatment. This involves either making or buying a finger splint. So, while you are completing your first week of baseline measurements, continue reading the next chapter as you may have some preparation to do before beginning your week 1 treatment which will follow week 0 (baseline diaries). Here are your first weeks' worth of diaries listed as week 0!

Trigger Finger Daily Diary		Week 0	Day 1
Date:		Modified SST score (see Key) 0-5	Pain Level (PNRS) (see key) 0-10
On waking after main sleep	At rest		
	On bending/straightening		
During most active period	At rest		
	On bending/straightening		
Just prior to main sleep	At rest		
	On bending/straightening		

Modified SST (stages of stenosing tenosynovitis) Score Key:

0	Normal finger movement
1	Uneven finger movement (looks smooth but feels rough)
2	Triggering or clicking or catching (looks a bit jerky, not fully smooth)
3	Finger locking in a bent or straight position but can unlock by active finger movements
4	Finger locking in a bent or straight position but unlocked by passive finger movements
5	Locked finger in bent or straightened position but cannot be unlocked at all

Pain Numeric Rating Scale (PNRS) Key

No pain 0 1 2 3 4 5 6 7 8 9 10 Worst pain Imaginable

My trigger finger today has:	Yes	No
Disturbed my sleep		
Prevented me from doing an activity I wanted or needed to do		
STATE AND DESCRIBE ACTIVITY:		

Medication for Trigger Finger: Frequency………………..times/day Medication Name: Total daily dose:	Yes	No
Can you make a full fist just before my main sleep?		
Can you straighten your fingers fully just before my main sleep?		

Trigger Finger Daily Diary		Week 0	Day 2
Date:		Modified SST score (see Key) 0-5	Pain Level (PNRS) (see key) 0-10
On waking after main sleep	At rest		
	On bending/straightening		
During most active period	At rest		
	On bending/straightening		
Just prior to main sleep	At rest		
	On bending/straightening		

Modified SST (stages of stenosing tenosynovitis) Score Key:

0 Normal finger movement
1 Uneven finger movement (looks smooth but feels rough)
2 Triggering or clicking or catching (looks a bit jerky, not fully smooth)
3 Finger locking in a bent or straight position but can unlock by active finger movements
4 Finger locking in a bent or straight position but unlocked by passive finger movements
5 Locked finger in bent or straightened position but cannot be unlocked at all

Pain Numeric Rating Scale (PNRS) Key

No pain 0 1 2 3 4 5 6 7 8 9 10 Worst pain imaginable

My trigger finger today has:	Yes	No
Disturbed my sleep		
Prevented me from doing an activity I wanted or needed to do STATE AND DESCRIBE ACTIVITY:		

Medication for Trigger Finger: Frequency.....................times/day Medication Name: Total daily dose:	Yes	No
Can you make a full fist just before main sleep?		
Can you straighten your fingers fully just before main sleep?		

Trigger Finger Daily Diary		Week 0	Day 3
Date:		Modified SST score (see Key) 0-5	Pain Level (PNRS) (see key) 0-10
On waking after main sleep	At rest		
	On bending/straightening		
During most active period	At rest		
	On bending/straightening		
Just prior to main sleep	At rest		
	On bending/straightening		

Modified SST (stages of stenosing tenosynovitis) Score Key:

0 Normal finger movement

1 Uneven finger movement (looks smooth but feels rough)

2 Triggering or clicking or catching (looks a bit jerky, not fully smooth)

3 Finger locking in a bent or straight position but can unlock by active finger movements

4 Finger locking in a bent or straight position but unlocked by passive finger movements

5 Locked finger in bent or straightened position but cannot be unlocked at all

Pain Numeric Rating Scale (PNRS) Key

No pain 0 1 2 3 4 5 6 7 8 9 10 Worst pain Imaginable

My trigger finger today has:	Yes	No
Disturbed my sleep		
Prevented me from doing an activity I wanted or needed to do		
STATE AND DESCRIBE ACTIVITY:		

Medication for Trigger Finger: Frequency....................times/day Medication Name: Total daily dose:	Yes	No
Can you make a full fist just before main sleep?		
Can you straighten your fingers fully just before main sleep?		

Trigger Finger Daily Diary		Week 0	Day 4
Date:		Modified SST score (see Key) 0-5	Pain Level (PNRS) (see key) 0-10
On waking after main sleep	At rest		
	On bending/straightening		
During most active period	At rest		
	On bending/straightening		
Just prior to main sleep	At rest		
	On bending/straightening		

Modified SST (stages of stenosing tenosynovitis) Score Key:

0 Normal finger movement
1 Uneven finger movement (looks smooth but feels rough)
2 Triggering or clicking or catching (looks a bit jerky, not fully smooth)
3 Finger locking in a bent or straight position but can unlock by active finger movements
4 Finger locking in a bent or straight position but unlocked by passive finger movements
5 Locked finger in bent or straightened position but cannot be unlocked at all

Pain Numeric Rating Scale (PNRS) Key

No pain											Worst pain Imaginable
	0	1	2	3	4	5	6	7	8	9	10

My trigger finger today has:	Yes	No
Disturbed my sleep		
Prevented me from doing an activity I wanted or needed to do STATE AND DESCRIBE ACTIVITY:		

Medication for Trigger Finger: Frequency.....................times/day Medication Name: Total daily dose:	Yes	No
Can you make a full fist just before main sleep?		
Can you straighten your fingers fully just before main sleep?		

Trigger Finger Daily Diary		Week 0	Day 5
Date:		Modified SST score (see Key) 0-5	Pain Level (PNRS) (see key) 0-10
On waking after main sleep	At rest		
	On bending/straightening		
During most active period	At rest		
	On bending/straightening		
Just prior to main sleep	At rest		
	On bending/straightening		

Modified SST (stages of stenosing tenosynovitis) Score Key:
0 Normal finger movement
1 Uneven finger movement (looks smooth but feels rough)
2 Triggering or clicking or catching (looks a bit jerky, not fully smooth)
3 Finger locking in a bent or straight position but can unlock by active finger movements
4 Finger locking in a bent or straight position but unlocked by passive finger movements
5 Locked finger in bent or straightened position but cannot be unlocked at all

Pain Numeric Rating Scale (PNRS) Key

No pain 0 1 2 3 4 5 6 7 8 9 10 Worst pain Imaginable

My trigger finger today has:	Yes	No
Disturbed my sleep		
Prevented me from doing an activity I wanted or needed to do STATE AND DESCRIBE ACTIVITY:		

Medication for Trigger Finger: Frequency....................times/day Medication Name: Total daily dose:	Yes	No
Can you make a full fist just before main sleep?		
Can you straighten your fingers fully just before main sleep?		

Trigger Finger Daily Diary		Week 0	Day 6
Date:		Modified SST score (see Key) 0-5	Pain Level (PNRS) (see key) 0-10
On waking after main sleep	At rest		
	On bending/straightening		
During most active period	At rest		
	On bending/straightening		
Just prior to main sleep	At rest		
	On bending/straightening		

Modified SST (stages of stenosing tenosynovitis) Score Key:
0 Normal finger movement
1 Uneven finger movement (looks smooth but feels rough)
2 Triggering or clicking or catching (looks a bit jerky, not fully smooth)
3 Finger locking in a bent or straight position but can unlock by active finger movements
4 Finger locking in a bent or straight position but unlocked by passive finger movements
5 Locked finger in bent or straightened position but cannot be unlocked at all

Pain Numeric Rating Scale (PNRS) Key

No pain 0 1 2 3 4 5 6 7 8 9 10 Worst pain Imaginable

My trigger finger today has:	Yes	No
Disturbed my sleep		
Prevented me from doing an activity I wanted or needed to do		
STATE AND DESCRIBE ACTIVITY:		

Medication for Trigger Finger: Frequency....................times/day Medication Name: Total daily dose:	Yes	No
Can you make a full fist just before main sleep?		
Can you straighten your fingers fully just before main sleep?		

Trigger Finger Daily Diary		Week 0	Day 7
Date:		Modified SST score (see Key) 0-5	Pain Level (PNRS) (see key) 0-10
On waking after main sleep	At rest		
	On bending/straightening		
During most active period	At rest		
	On bending/straightening		
Just prior to main sleep	At rest		
	On bending/straightening		

Modified SST (stages of stenosing tenosynovitis) Score Key:

0 Normal finger movement
1 Uneven finger movement (looks smooth but feels rough)
2 Triggering or clicking or catching (looks a bit jerky, not fully smooth)
3 Finger locking in a bent or straight position but can unlock by active finger movements
4 Finger locking in a bent or straight position but unlocked by passive finger movements
5 Locked finger in bent or straightened position but cannot be unlocked at all

Pain Numeric Rating Scale (PNRS) Key

No pain 0 1 2 3 4 5 6 7 8 9 10 Worst pain Imaginable

My trigger finger today has:	Yes	No
Disturbed my sleep		
Prevented me from doing an activity I wanted or needed to do STATE AND DESCRIBE ACTIVITY:		

Medication for Trigger Finger: Frequency....................times/day Medication Name: Total daily dose:	Yes	No
Can you make a full fist just before main sleep?		
Can you straighten your fingers fully just before main sleep?		

Chapter 3: Week 1: 1st Treatment – Finger Splints

A finger splint is simply a rigid or semi-rigid board which can be made of anything from a piece of plastic or wood and even something which has been bought 'off the shelf' through a to bespoke 'made to measure' device fashioned by an expert orthotist or hand therapist. The photos (photos 3, 4, 5 and 6) below show you an example of an 'off the self' finger splint. I would advise the use of this type of bought, 'off the shelf' sort of splint simply because it is easy to don and doff (put on and take off). It is also easy to keep clean, inexpensive and comfortable to wear. In Appendix 1, I show you how you can make your own splint but with this, comes some disadvantages: Firstly, they are awkward to make at the best of times but when you have some hand dysfunction (such as trigger finger) the problem is augmented. Secondly, gathering the materials isn't always convenient although often people have them lying around (as I did). Thirdly, they are more difficult to keep clean and fourthly, they tend to be more rigid and therefore less comfortable. Finally, they are more difficult to don and doff and when they are applied too tightly, they can be problematic to the body's circulation, causing the finger to discolour, go numb or become too painful to wear, requiring the whole thing to be removed. This latter point is also true of the 'off the shelf' type, but these are far more easily adjusted.

However, all that said, there will be those readers who are naturally good at 'craft' and would welcome the challenge of making their own splint or, better still, they may know someone, a friend or relative perhaps, who would make one for then. I would not want to stand in the way of thrift and creativity so essentially the choice is yours. However, before doing this, please take a look at the advice given in Appendix 1 regarding some basic principles and safety advice.

So, to begin with, let's take a look at the 'off the shelf' splint and consider what it looks like and how you apply it. Photos 3a and b show the front and back views respectively of a typical kind of 'bought' splint. I bought this one on-line for just a few pounds. Normally, they arrive within a few days but there can he hold-ups so it is best to order it now, and while you are reading the rest of this chapter (and most of the next) you can wait for its arrival. The splint is easy to apply and take off and can be easily adjusted in the event that initially it is put on too tightly.

Photo 3: a and b Example of an 'off the shelf' Finger Splint

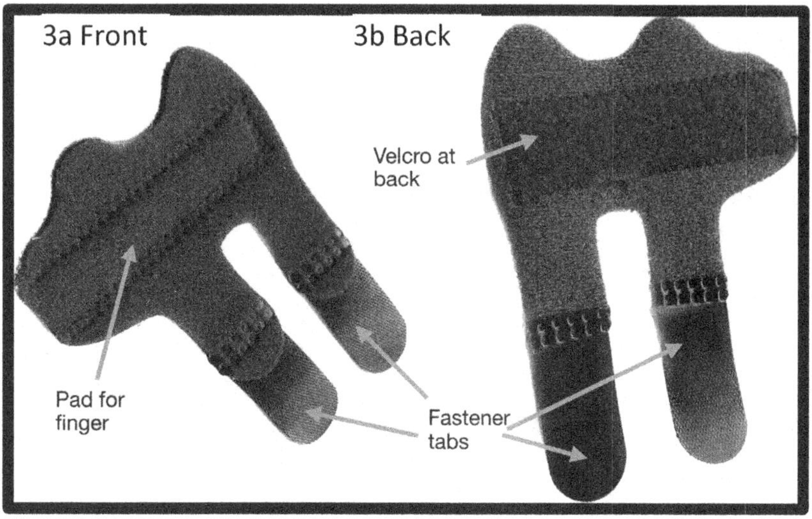

Photos 4a and 4b show how to apply the splint. This can be a bit fiddly to begin with but you soon get the knack. The best way is to lie the splint on it back and to then place the affected finger of the pad. Then, take the tab furthest away from the hand and tie that on first to anchor the splint. Then, tie the tab closest to the palm. If you would like to see a video of me putting on this splint, go to this link:

https://www.youtube.com/watch?v=g81Ri2qHgsQ

Photo 4: a and b Application of 'off the shelf' Finger Splint

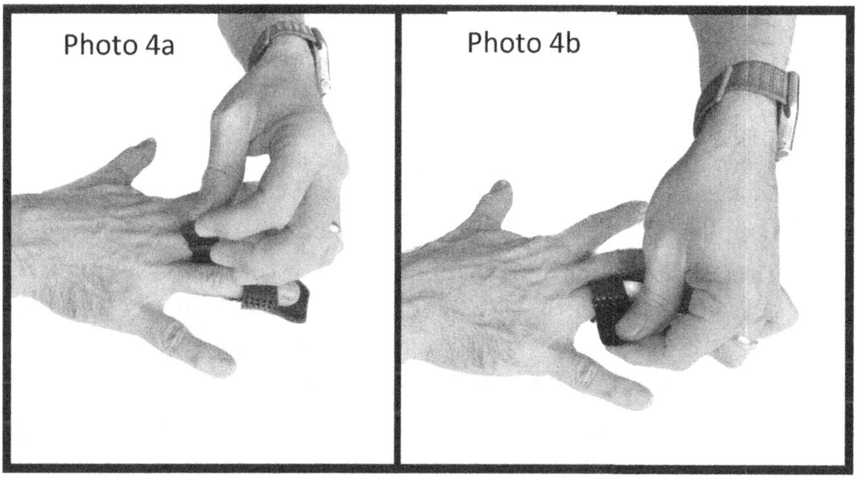

Photos 5a and 5b show the front (palmar) and rear (dorsal) aspects of the splint once it has been applied. However, photos 5a and 5b show an alternative application.

Photo 5: a and b Use of an 'off the shelf' finger splint

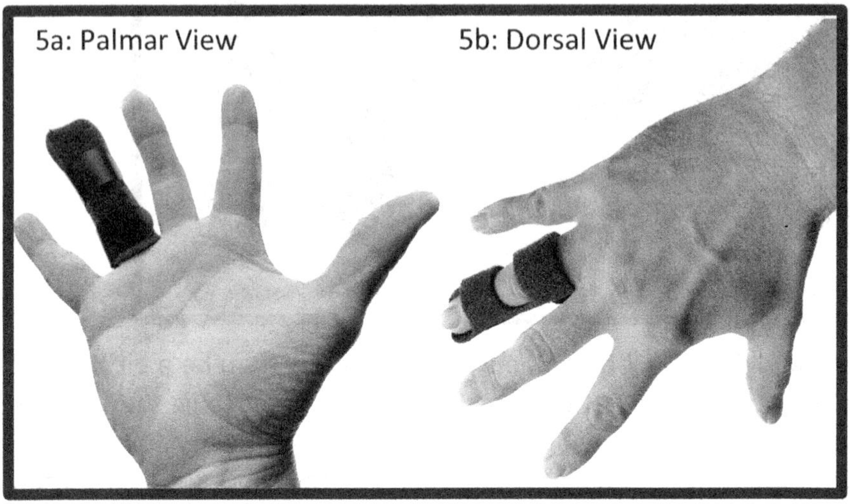

The problem with the application shown in photos 5a and 5b, is that one of the observed characteristics of trigger finger, is that at night, the hand tends to want to curl into a fist. This is not always the case, but in a large number of people who have trigger finger, this does appear to be so. As you can see, from photo 5b, that in the night, if a fist is formed, it is possible that the splint will not prevent this completely and might make it more difficult, and likely as not, more uncomfortable to wear because the curling finger will strain against the straps, thus increasing the tightness of the splint. Under these circumstances, it is likely that the wearer, probably half asleep, will rip the splint off.

This, half conscious, night-time removal of the splint can be a problem even if the splint is applied in the way described in photos 6a and 6b, however, it is less likely as this is a more comfortable way to wear a splint at night. It should also be said that wearing a splint is something that needs to be practised before it is used in earnest. The best way to do this, is to initially wear the splint during the day, during periods of rest so that you get used to using it. Only then, when you are completely comfortable and well-practised with its use, should you apply it at night.

Photo 6: a and b Alternative Application of an 'off the shelf' Finger Splint

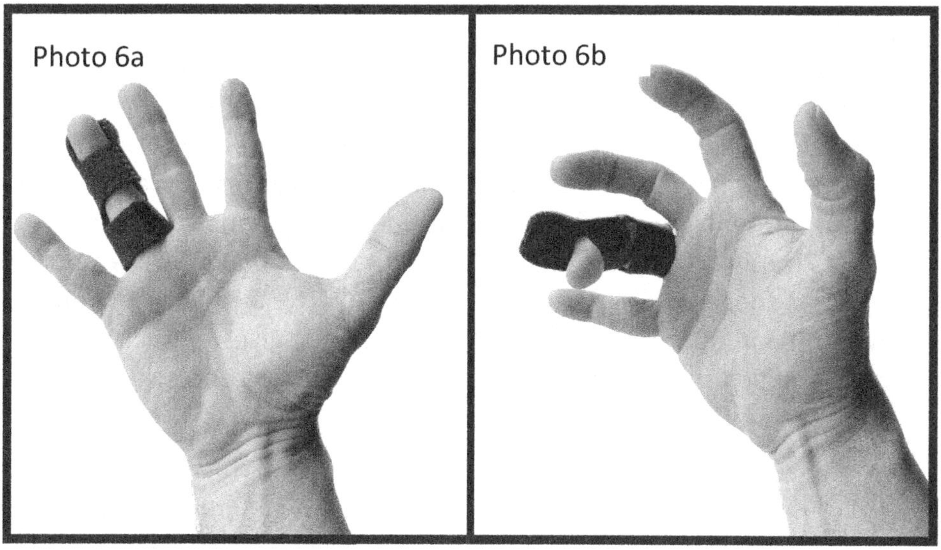

Okay, so what else do you need to know about splints? Well, in this chapter, I will also tell you the best way to use this finger splint and what wearing a finger splint might tell you about our trigger finger. This first week of treatment (following 7-days of just measuring with no intervention) explores the use of a finger splint. Many people reading this book will have already tried this. However, I want to come at it from a slightly different angle. First of all, we can use a finger splint to tell us something about the nature of **our** trigger finger.

For example, although there is no certainty about whether or not trigger finger is caused by inflammation, there is no doubt there is clearly mechanical dysfunction which brings about a change in movement of the finger: triggering, locking, uneven movement etc. Pain can occur in trigger finger at different times. For example, some people complain of constant pain in the hand, even at rest but when they bend their fingers and it "triggers" the pain spikes at the point of triggering or locking or whatever. In this scenario, people often avoid making a fist or performing gripping activities because the hand is painful all the time and so they avoid spiking the pain which can be so severe that people can visibly wince. These people are in the greatest danger of having a permanently locked finger and regressing to a grade 6 on the SST scale together with hand muscle atrophy (wasting).

Pain can be intermittent, meaning that sometimes it can be present and sometimes not. Whether or not the pain is present is often related to the nature of things that have been done with the hand. For example, it would not be uncommon for somebody using hand tools, such as shovels, spades, shears for gardening, to feel no pain during the gardening process, but, later that evening, the hand may ache and feel as though it is gradually stiffening as the evening progresses. This would be a sign of low grade, chronic inflammation. In this case, movement gives sufficient local lubrication which masks the physical irritation but rest encourages latent fluid reabsorption and tissue binding.

When a hand with trigger finger is constantly painful (even at rest) this normally indicates that an acute inflammatory reaction is taking place however, we cannot say for certain why and where the inflammation is. When there is no pain at rest, but there is pain on activity, which ceases once the activity is stopped, it is **unlikely** that the root of the trigger finger is inflammatory but rather more likely to be mechanically stimulated pain. When people have pain most of the time and this spikes on movement and in particular triggering or locking, this means that there is both a combination of inflammatory and mechanical pain taking place. We don't need to understand the detailed distinction between the inflammatory pain and mechanical pain here as this is covered fully in my other book on the ManTTr® Protocol[5]. However, we do need to consider for a moment what benefits the use of a splints would be in determining whether or not the pain is inflammatory, mechanical or both.

Although splints can be used for a number of things, the most common reason splints are used is to provide rest and to some extent, protection. The protection element, is to avoid excessive use of the compromised body part and also to prevent it from being further irritated or aggravated. As a method of producing enforced rest, the splint provides time for the cardinal signs of the tissue repair cascade, and in particular its inflammatory element, to subside. There are four main "cardinal" signs of inflammation and these are: redness, swelling, pain, and heat. In severe cases, a 5th sign of loss of function (which is really an aggregation of the 4 main signs) is also included. This latter point may or may not be the case for trigger finger.

Under normal healing conditions, these cardinal signs initially erupt at the time of the injury, irritation or damage, peaking at around 12 hours[51]. Then, over a period of days and weeks, the cellular activity associated with them subsides and the cardinal signs diminish, ending in resolution at which point there are only residual signs such as tenderness, and in some cases, scarring remaining. Under circumstances where pain is constant in trigger finger and/ or there is constant pain together with a spiking of pain on movement, we tend to presume that the underlying problem is inflammatory. If we continue to use the hand, it is possible that this inflammation is being perpetuated by aberrant forces caused by the hand's continued use. In order to stop these aberrant forces and/or any other forces acting to perpetuating inflammation, we can rest the trigger finger and the best way to do this is in a splint.

The reason a splint is used, and not something more solid like plaster of Paris or other, more contemporary, materials for retaining body parts, is because we need to make sure that the finger is able to move through its full range of motion at least twice a day to avoid stiffness from setting in. This means that we have to be able to remove the retaining structure, in this case the splint. In this way, the splint acts to protect from aberrant forces and also allows the finger to rest. However, as previously stated, it must not rest permanently as learned disuse will cause stiffness and so we must take it out of the splint twice a day to move the finger under a degree of control and minimise the effect of the triggering. It is hoped that by doing this, the finger will be given sufficient time for the inflammatory processes to complete and therefore allow for shrinkage of thickened or swollen tissue in and around the A1 pulley.

However, it is unlikely that this intervention will bring about a miraculous change in the state of your trigger finger mainly because it takes a great many months for thickened tissues to shrink, although it is possible that swelling may reduce in a relatively short period of time. Most people who have used splints in the past have been unsuccessful in solving their trigger finger problem because they have not allowed sufficient time for it to have its effect and, they have also used it in isolation and not in combination with other forms of therapy to complement and augment its use. That said, it is an important step to take because, at this point in our self-treatment, we are not sure about your trigger finger inflammatory status. We also don't know what activities or functions that may be perpetuating your symptoms. To that end, wearing a splint might help us to gain additional information about the status of your trigger finger. If you find that by wearing a splint, your pain levels go down, then this indicates that movement around the triggering site is causing pain and so it is likely that your pain is mainly mechanical. If you find that the pain remains steady, possibly with some diminution in discomfort, this might suggest that your problem is mainly inflammatory. So, in this latter case, with some prolonged and judicious use of a splint in combination with some other techniques that I will show you later in the book, the splint is likely to contribute, at least in some way, to you making progress with your trigger finger symptoms. However, it should be noted that the objective of the strategies included in this book is aimed at getting rid of the need for a finger splint and for your hand to return to normal, or close to normal functioning.

You can see from the photos 3-6 above that a trigger finger splint is a very simple device and Appendix 1 shows how it can be fashioned from the simplest of materials. However, I would recommend that you bought a ready-made 'off the peg' splint. Obviously, this costs more money but in the scheme of things, it is a very small amount to pay. The reason that I suggest this, is that it is designed in such a way as to allow you to have some movement but certainly not enough to cause a problem to the joints most affected by a trigger finger. Making your own splint out of a piece of plastic, or perhaps even a lolly stick, tied on with medical tape will do the job, but they will not have as much comfort and will require that you take precautions such as testing to see if you are allergic to that particular kind of tape and also wearing a finger cover over the splint so that you do not inadvertently poke yourself in the face or some other body part while wearing the splint. Then again, the bottom line for wearing a finger splint is that it keeps your finger still for prolonged periods and that it does so safely... that is all that is required!

It is difficult to give you specific advice about using a finger splint other than to say that you need to be pragmatic and use it when you can in addition to the night-time. For example, if you are a touch typist and you are wearing a finger splint, you are going to find it very difficult to type and so you should refrain from wearing it when doing that activity. However, during other periods, for example, when reading or filing or doing some other clerical activity, it might be possible to function perfectly well and safely with the finger in the splint. On the other side of the coin, if you are a manual worker, it might be difficult to wear a splint if you are handling tools which could be potentially dangerous if you did not have full control of them, in which case you would need to remove the splint for that purpose. However, during down time for, example breaks and when at home and at night when you are in bed, there is no reason why you should not have the splint in position.

The balance between when to and when not to use a splint (otherwise referred to as an orthotic) is one of the regimen issues identified in the literature[52]. In theory they are practicable if you can incorporate them into a daily routine and if so, may provide your finger with adequate rest, and in so doing, may provide you with a better than evens chance of reducing some of your symptoms. However, the chances of it fixing the problem are remote unless you can commit to its use for around 1 year when you will have about a 66% chance of fixing the problem[11]. That said, we need to see the use of the splints within the context of this book as merely one slice of the pie. It's a relatively small slice at that, but it is nonetheless a worthwhile thing to begin with.

In terms of the duration of having your finger in the splint, this should be for no longer than eight hours at a time. After that amount of time, you should take your splint off and move your hand through its full range of motion slowly and deliberately, taking care not to do anything rapid or something that will cause hand pain, if this is at all avoidable as this can reignite the local inflammatory reaction that we are trying to subdue. Although I have advised against the use of anti-inflammatory agents and painkillers, there is no reason why they cannot be used in conjunction with splinting if you are able, permitted and wish to.

So, let's think where we are now: while you are reading this section of the book, you are contemplating the application of a splint for your finger. You are also filling out your baseline diary which is the current state of your trigger finger over a seven-day period in the absence of doing any interventions. On day 8, you will start using the splint and during that time you will complete a second daily diary (Week 1 diary). So, I now need to talk to you about the second treatment that I would like you to include after you've completed one week of only applying the splint. In the third week of diaries (Week 2 diary) I would like you to bathe your elbow, forearm, wrist and hand in warm water. Figure 5 below provides an outline of activities to be concluded within the first 3 weeks.

Figure 5: Summary of Progress to Week 1

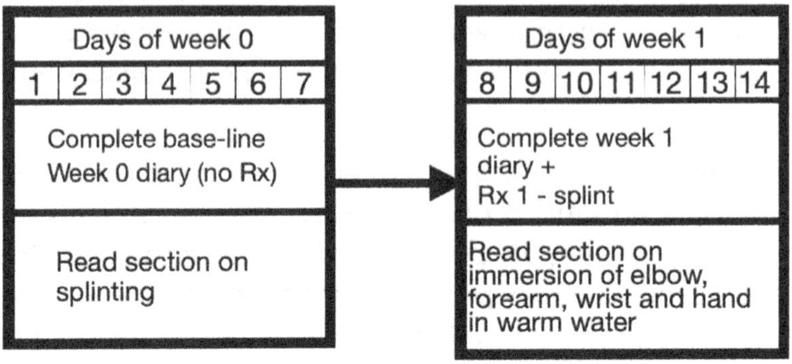

Rx=Treatment

So, next, here are your Week 1 diaries. Now that you have completed Week 0 Diaries, you should be familiar with the measurement scales. So, you should not need the modified SST and PNRS scale keys each day, so I will only provide you with a key to each scale at the start of the week and then provide an abbreviated diary:

Week 1 Diaries

Modified SST (stages of stenosing tenosynovitis) Score Key:
0 Normal finger movement
1 Uneven finger movement (looks smooth but feels rough)
2 Triggering or clicking or catching (looks a bit jerky, not fully smooth)
3 Finger locking in a bent or straight position but can unlock by active finger movements
4 Finger locking in a bent or straight position but unlocked by passive finger movements
5 Locked finger in bent or straightened position but cannot be unlocked at all
Pain Numeric Rating Scale (PNRS) Key:
No pain 0 1 2 3 4 5 6 7 8 9 10 Worst pain imaginable

Trigger Finger Daily Diary		Week 1 Day 1	
Date:		Modified SST score (see Key) 0-5	Pain Level (PNRS) (see key) 0-10
On waking after main sleep	At rest		
	On bending/straightening		
During most active period	At rest		
	On bending/straightening		
Just prior to main sleep	At rest		
	On bending/straightening		

My trigger finger today has:	Yes	No
Disturbed my sleep		
Prevented me from doing an activity I wanted or needed to do		
STATE AND DESCRIBE ACTIVITY:		
Medication for Trigger Finger: Frequency...................times/day **Medication Name: Total daily dose:**	Yes	No
Can you make a full fist just before my main sleep?		
Can you straighten your fingers fully just before my main sleep?		

Trigger Finger Daily Diary		Week 1 Day 2	
Date:		Modified SST score (see Key) 0-5	Pain Level (PNRS) (see key) 0-10
On waking after main sleep	At rest		
	On bending/straightening		
During most active period	At rest		
	On bending/straightening		
Just prior to main sleep	At rest		
	On bending/straightening		

My trigger finger today has:	Yes	No
Disturbed my sleep		
Prevented me from doing an activity I wanted or needed to do		
STATE AND DESCRIBE ACTIVITY:		
Medication for Trigger Finger: Frequency...................times/day **Medication Name: Total daily dose:**	Yes	No
Can you make a full fist just before my main sleep?		
Can you straighten your fingers fully just before my main sleep?		

Trigger Finger Daily Diary		Week 1 Day 3	
Date:		Modified SST score (see Key) 0-5	Pain Level (PNRS) (see key) 0-10
On waking after main sleep	At rest		
	On bending/straightening		
During most active period	At rest		
	On bending/straightening		
Just prior to main sleep	At rest		
	On bending/straightening		
My trigger finger today has:		Yes	No
Disturbed my sleep			
Prevented me from doing an activity I wanted or needed to do STATE AND DESCRIBE ACTIVITY:			
Medication for Trigger Finger: Frequency……………….times/day Medication Name: Total daily dose:		Yes	No
Can you make a full fist just before my main sleep?			
Can you straighten your fingers fully just before my main sleep?			

Trigger Finger Daily Diary		Week 1 Day 4	
Date:		Modified SST score (see Key) 0-5	Pain Level (PNRS) (see key) 0-10
On waking after main sleep	At rest		
	On bending/straightening		
During most active period	At rest		
	On bending/straightening		
Just prior to main sleep	At rest		
	On bending/straightening		
My trigger finger today has:		Yes	No
Disturbed my sleep			
Prevented me from doing an activity I wanted or needed to do STATE AND DESCRIBE ACTIVITY:			
Medication for Trigger Finger: Frequency……………….times/day Medication Name: Total daily dose:		Yes	No
Can you make a full fist just before my main sleep?			
Can you straighten your fingers fully just before my main sleep?			

Trigger Finger Daily Diary		Week 1	Day 5	
Date:		Modified SST score (see Key) 0-5	Pain Level (PNRS) (see key) 0-10	
On waking after main sleep	At rest			
	On bending/straightening			
During most active period	At rest			
	On bending/straightening			
Just prior to main sleep	At rest			
	On bending/straightening			
My trigger finger today has:			Yes	No
Disturbed my sleep				
Prevented me from doing an activity I wanted or needed to do STATE AND DESCRIBE ACTIVITY:				
Medication for Trigger Finger: Frequency………………..times/day Medication Name: Total daily dose:			Yes	No
Can you make a full fist just before my main sleep?				
Can you straighten your fingers fully just before my main sleep?				

Trigger Finger Daily Diary		Week 1	Day 6	
Date:		Modified SST score (see Key) 0-5	Pain Level (PNRS) (see key) 0-10	
On waking after main sleep	At rest			
	On bending/straightening			
During most active period	At rest			
	On bending/straightening			
Just prior to main sleep	At rest			
	On bending/straightening			
My trigger finger today has:			Yes	No
Disturbed my sleep				
Prevented me from doing an activity I wanted or needed to do STATE AND DESCRIBE ACTIVITY:				
Medication for Trigger Finger: Frequency………………..times/day Medication Name: Total daily dose:			Yes	No
Can you make a full fist just before my main sleep?				
Can you straighten your fingers fully just before my main sleep?				

Trigger Finger Daily Diary	Week 1 Day 7	

Date:		Modified SST score (see Key) 0-5	Pain Level (PNRS) (see key) 0-10
On waking after main sleep	At rest		
	On bending/straightening		
During most active period	At rest		
	On bending/straightening		
Just prior to main sleep	At rest		
	On bending/straightening		

My trigger finger today has:	Yes	No
Disturbed my sleep		
Prevented me from doing an activity I wanted or needed to do		
STATE AND DESCRIBE ACTIVITY:		

Medication for Trigger Finger: Frequency....................times/day Medication Name: Total daily dose:	Yes	No
Can you make a full fist just before my main sleep?		
Can you straighten your fingers fully just before my main sleep?		

Chapter 4: Week 2, 2nd Treatment: Warm Water Immersion

Considering Figure 5 towards the end of the previous chapter, you will notice that the second week of treatment is about the immersion of your elbow, forearm, wrist and hand in warm water. I suspect there will be many wondering why, when the problem is in finger, we need to be so anatomically extensive with our heating. This is a very good point and requires some explanation! Naturally, I'm sure you are already aware, that this explanation is given in full in my book describing and demonstrating the ManTTr® Protocol[5] but, for the sake of this self-help book, which is much more concise than my book on the ManTTr® Protocol[5], I will give you a sufficient but unfortunately necessary superficial explanation. The fact is, that the tendons that are affected by trigger finger in the hand are actually positioned in the forearm. The highest points at which one of these muscles attaches is just above the elbow. The names of these muscles are *flexor digitorum superficialis* and *flexor digitorum profundus*. All this Latin nomenclature is quite confusing but if I may, just for a moment, explain what these Latin words actually mean, it will be less confusing:

To 'flex' a body part is, generally speaking, another word for bending a joint. Commonly, if you described somebody who is flexible, then it is as likely as not that you would be describing their ability to bend their body in various ways... they would have a 'bendy' body. The opposite to "flex" this is to "extend". So, if I flex my fingers, I bend them and if I extend my fingers, it means that I straighten them. This is not always an accurate description of what goes on throughout the body because there are some exceptions to this, however we are going to ignore them as they are not relevant to our subject matter. Generally, though, when a muscle is described as a 'flexor', it normally bends something in the body. *Digitorum* refers to the digits and that can mean the toes or the fingers. *Profundus* means deep (c.f. profound) and *superficialis* means superficial so you would expect that *flexor digitorum superficialis* is superficial to *flexor digitorum profundus* and you would be right, one (*superficialis*) lies directly over the other (*profundus*).

Confusion between the flexors and extensors of the toes and the fingers is avoided by the fact that in the arm the finger flexors are known as *profundus* and *superficialis* but the equivalent muscles in the leg that flex the toes, are known as *longus* (long) and *brevis* (short). So, if we interpret the name *flexor digitorum profundus*, this means the 'deep finger bender'. *Flexor digitorum superficialis* means the 'superficial finger bender'. These are the only muscles that bend the fingers whose muscle bellies are situated in the forearm. All of the other muscles that bend the fingers are situated in the hand. For this reason, *flexor digitorum profundus* (FDP) and *flexor digitorum superficialis* (FDS) are together known as the 'extrinsic finger flexors'. This is very important for trigger finger because the tendons of these two muscles are those that get stuck in the A1 pulley when the fingers are bent (flexed) or straightened (extended). As such, the relative length and flexibility of the extrinsic flexors may have an influence on the position of the tendons in the hand. If, having developed trigger finger, we ignore the position and state of the extrinsic finger flexors, we are missing an important element which might positively influence the biomechanics in the hand.

As such, the rationale behind the immersion of the whole of the elbow, forearm, wrist and hand in the water is so that the heat is able to sufficiently, and evenly penetrate ALL of the tissues in the forearm including the muscles, ligaments, tendons, nerves, blood vessels, lymph channels and other soft tissues including the fascia (which is a ubiquitous tissue constructed mainly of the protein collagen, connecting everything to everything else). Heating also has a pain killing effect which allows us to move painful areas more easily and comfortably. The type of heating that we are trying to apply cannot be achieved by placing a hot water bottle or hot pack or such like on the various target areas. Only the complete immersion in warm water will be able to do this.

The application of heat is particularly useful when mobilising tissues[53]. This is because it creates suppleness and pliability in the tissues allowing them to elongate more easily when they are stretched. It also increases the local blood supply in the immersed areas which, in turn, assists in facilitating healing, should that be required. Heating should not be used if there are open wounds and if there is internal bleeding in the limb. This is because heat will slow down and even interrupt the clotting process and perpetuate bleeding, thus hindering the wound healing cascade. People with sensation deficits or hyper-sensitivity should also exercise caution and always measure the temperature of the water very accurately by using a correctly calibrated thermometer.

Immersing the elbow, forearm, wrist and hand into water is relatively straightforward as a simple kitchen sink can be used (see Photos 7 and 8). The temperature of the water should feel comfortable and not too hot. Temperatures around 38^0 C (100.4^0 F) should be adequate as this is just above the temperature of the human body which is around 37^0 C (98.6^0F). It would be wise to measure this temperature and test it with the back of your hand just prior to immersing the elbow, forearm, wrist and hand. Some people may prefer higher temperatures but this is NOT a case of higher temperature is better. The water need only feel comfortably warm and should NOT feel hot!

While immersed, you should, after a couple of minutes, begin to bend and straighten the fingers initially doing so just short of triggering the finger. However, over a period of 10 minutes, you should aim to be able to make a complete fist and full straightening of the fingers at least 10 times while you are immersed in the water. Ideally, this should be done at the start of the day to allow the fingers to use the pliability for functional activities. This activity should be undertaken twice a day, with the 2nd of the two immersions being at the end of the working day. This exercise regimen should be continued for many weeks or even months.

Photo 7:Immersion of Forearm and Hand in Warm Water - Flexion

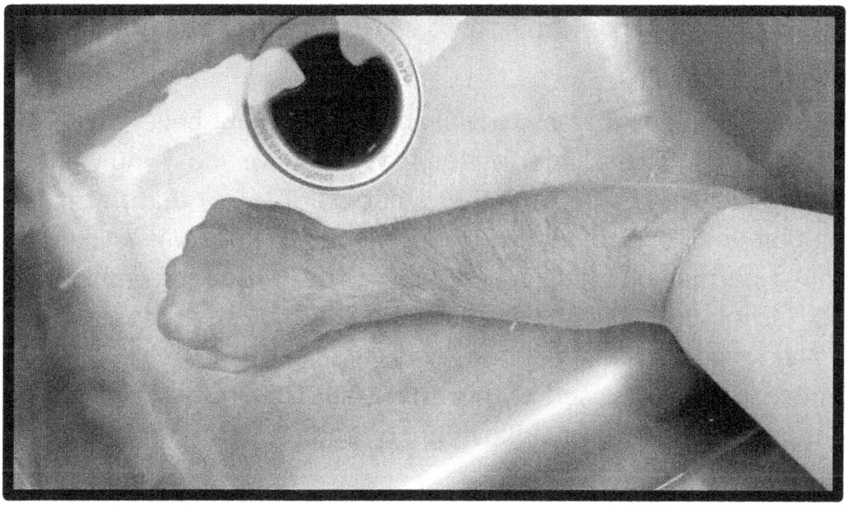

Photo 8: Immersion of Forearm and Hand in Warm Water - Extension

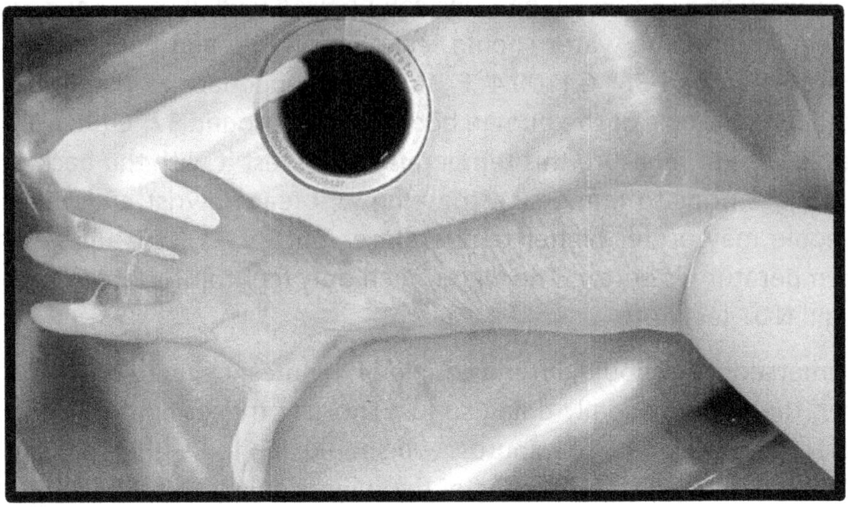

One of the biggest drawbacks to conducting this water regimen is that people find it boring. Some people don't like the fact that the warm water makes the skin wrinkle and others complain that it dries the skin. These latter two things have simple remedies which is to moisturise the hand after it has been thoroughly dried after the immersion. The solution for boredom lies in effective distraction. I usually advise people to pick three tunes from their music list and to play them. Bearing in mind that most songs these days are in the region of three minutes in duration, after three tunes there is only around one minute to wait before you can remove your hand from the water.

This exercise might appear rather trivial and pointless but believe me, it is the most important piece of information that I can give you if you want to overcome the problem of trigger finger. That is not to say that this is the only thing that you need to do as only applying this strategy is unlikely to bring about a permanent change. However, if this is used in combination with other techniques, which I will show you soon, it can produce one of the best and longest lasting solutions to trigger finger. I should say that water immersion is also used within the ManTTr® Protocol[5], not as a primary treatment, but as a follow up treatment after the ManTTr® Protocol[5] has been applied.

So, let's take a look at where we are now. If things are going to schedule, you will be using your finger splint at night and you will have read what is coming up next. So, after you've completed your week of using the splint, you will then begin a new 7-day diary only this time, you will add in the regimen of immersion in warm water. During that week, you will read about what comes next, and that is: tendon elongation/gliding/stretching.

Figure 6: Summary of Progress to Week 2

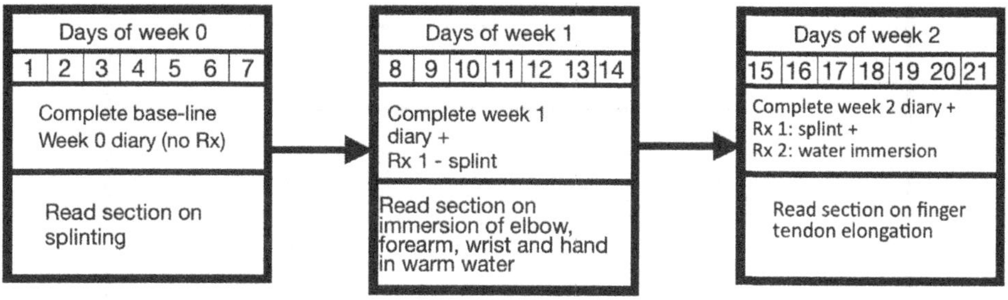

Week 2 Diaries

Modified SST (stages of stenosing tenosynovitis) Score Key:
0 Normal finger movement
1 Uneven finger movement (looks smooth but feels rough)
2 Triggering or clicking or catching (looks a bit jerky, not fully smooth)
3 Finger locking in a bent or straight position but can unlock by active finger movements
4 Finger locking in a bent or straight position but unlocked by passive finger movements
5 Locked finger in bent or straightened position but cannot be unlocked at all
Pain Numeric Rating Scale (PNRS) Key:

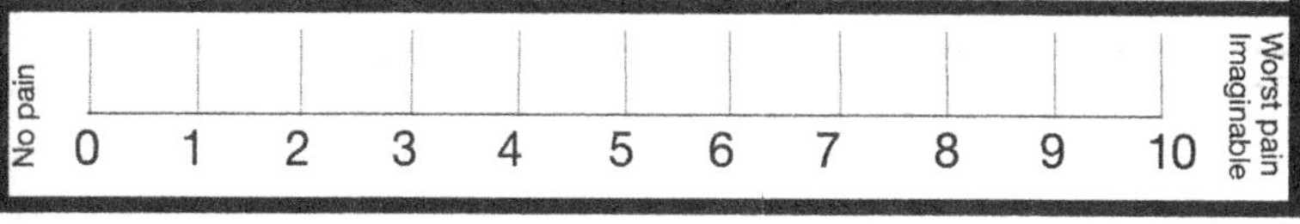

Trigger Finger Daily Diary		Week 2 Day 1	
Date:		Modified SST score (see Key) 0-5	Pain Level (PNRS) (see key) 0-10
On waking after main sleep	At rest		
	On bending/straightening		
During most active period	At rest		
	On bending/straightening		
Just prior to main sleep	At rest		
	On bending/straightening		

My trigger finger today has:	Yes	No
Disturbed my sleep		
Prevented me from doing an activity I wanted or needed to do STATE AND DESCRIBE ACTIVITY:		
Medication for Trigger Finger: Frequency....................times/day Medication Name: Total daily dose:	Yes	No
Can you make a full fist just before my main sleep?		
Can you straighten your fingers fully just before my main sleep?		

Trigger Finger Daily Diary		Week 2 Day 2	
Date:		Modified SST score (see Key) 0-5	Pain Level (PNRS) (see key) 0-10
On waking after main sleep	At rest		
	On bending/straightening		
During most active period	At rest		
	On bending/straightening		
Just prior to main sleep	At rest		
	On bending/straightening		

My trigger finger today has:	Yes	No
Disturbed my sleep		
Prevented me from doing an activity I wanted or needed to do STATE AND DESCRIBE ACTIVITY:		
Medication for Trigger Finger: Frequency....................times/day Medication Name: Total daily dose:	Yes	No
Can you make a full fist just before my main sleep?		
Can you straighten your fingers fully just before my main sleep?		

Trigger Finger Daily Diary		Week 2 Day 3	
Date:		Modified SST score (see Key) 0-5	Pain Level (PNRS) (see key) 0-10
On waking after main sleep	At rest		
	On bending/straightening		
During most active period	At rest		
	On bending/straightening		
Just prior to main sleep	At rest		
	On bending/straightening		

My trigger finger today has:	Yes	No
Disturbed my sleep		
Prevented me from doing an activity I wanted or needed to do		
STATE AND DESCRIBE ACTIVITY:		
Medication for Trigger Finger: Frequency………………..times/day Medication Name: Total daily dose:	Yes	No
Can you make a full fist just before my main sleep?		
Can you straighten your fingers fully just before my main sleep?		

Trigger Finger Daily Diary		Week 2 Day 4	
Date:		Modified SST score (see Key) 0-5	Pain Level (PNRS) (see key) 0-10
On waking after main sleep	At rest		
	On bending/straightening		
During most active period	At rest		
	On bending/straightening		
Just prior to main sleep	At rest		
	On bending/straightening		

My trigger finger today has:	Yes	No
Disturbed my sleep		
Prevented me from doing an activity I wanted or needed to do		
STATE AND DESCRIBE ACTIVITY:		
Medication for Trigger Finger: Frequency………………..times/day Medication Name: Total daily dose:	Yes	No
Can you make a full fist just before my main sleep?		
Can you straighten your fingers fully just before my main sleep?		

Trigger Finger Daily Diary		Week 2 Day 5	
Date:		Modified SST score (see Key) 0-5	Pain Level (PNRS) (see key) 0-10
On waking after main sleep	At rest		
	On bending/straightening		
During most active period	At rest		
	On bending/straightening		
Just prior to main sleep	At rest		
	On bending/straightening		

My trigger finger today has:	Yes	No
Disturbed my sleep		
Prevented me from doing an activity I wanted or needed to do		
STATE AND DESCRIBE ACTIVITY:		

Medication for Trigger Finger: Frequency....................times/day Medication Name: Total daily dose:	Yes	No
Can you make a full fist just before my main sleep?		
Can you straighten your fingers fully just before my main sleep?		

Trigger Finger Daily Diary		Week 2 Day 6	
Date:		Modified SST score (see Key) 0-5	Pain Level (PNRS) (see key) 0-10
On waking after main sleep	At rest		
	On bending/straightening		
During most active period	At rest		
	On bending/straightening		
Just prior to main sleep	At rest		
	On bending/straightening		

My trigger finger today has:	Yes	No
Disturbed my sleep		
Prevented me from doing an activity I wanted or needed to do		
STATE AND DESCRIBE ACTIVITY:		

Medication for Trigger Finger: Frequency....................times/day Medication Name: Total daily dose:	Yes	No
Can you make a full fist just before my main sleep?		
Can you straighten your fingers fully just before my main sleep?		

Trigger Finger Daily Diary		Week 2 Day 7	
Date:		Modified SST score (see Key) 0-5	Pain Level (PNRS) (see key) 0-10
On waking after main sleep	At rest		
	On bending/straightening		
During most active period	At rest		
	On bending/straightening		
Just prior to main sleep	At rest		
	On bending/straightening		

My trigger finger today has:	Yes	No
Disturbed my sleep		
Prevented me from doing an activity I wanted or needed to do		
STATE AND DESCRIBE ACTIVITY:		

Medication for Trigger Finger: Frequency.....................times/day Medication Name: Total daily dose:	Yes	No
Can you make a full fist just before my main sleep?		
Can you straighten your fingers fully just before my main sleep?		

Chapter 5: Week 3, 3rd Treatment: Tendon Elongation

Well, I hope you have been able to stick to the programme so far and you're not jumping the gun! If you do jump the gun, that is, if you do things in the wrong order or you rushed to do everything all at once, the chance of success will not be as good as they otherwise would be. Don't forget, that it is just as important that you accurately record your journey and that you engage in a measured and progressive manner. The other thing that you need to bear in mind is that if you are racing ahead more rapidly than you should, there is a far higher chance that you will create aggravation and even greater pain. As such, it is absolutely imperative that you stick to the timing and the chronology of the suggested measurements and interventions. The reason for this is that with every intervention that is made, there is a slight change to your body which then needs time to adjust to this new situation by recalibrating itself and to cope with any imposed change. Overloading the body too rapidly using the techniques shown in this book results in a failure to recalibrate and further structural dysfunction.

You will notice that I have underlined some words in the previous paragraph, specifically "using the techniques shown in this book." The reason I have done this is because there are techniques which bring about a rapid change in the state of trigger finger. These are described in the ManTTr® Protocol[5]but this approach can only be undertaken by a skilled practitioner. Even with the ManTTr® Protocol[5], there are sometimes side effects which cause a temporary increase in discomfort all of which can be dealt with by subsidiary treatment. This subsidiary treatment, however, can only be conducted and supervised by suitably qualified third parties. Even in the ManTTr® Protocol[5] the body has to be given time to recalibrate for the changes created to the biomechanics which, I believe, are the cause of trigger finger in the first place. All of this is explained in my book on the ManTTr® Protocol[5] which, is a guide for therapists and an educational source for people who have trigger finger or an interest in trigger finger.

Now, having clarified this point, returning to the self-treatment approach: You may have noticed that the first two treatments that I have suggested to you are generally palliative (aims to reduce symptoms) and non-aggravating. The splint is there to allow the finger to rest and the exercise in water is a means by which you can make the tissues more supple and allow for mobility of the tissues without creating any aggravation. These are also treatments that you can use during times when your hand is particularly uncomfortable as both aim to reduce pain in a non-chemical way. The next two interventions that you will do, will be different from the point of view that they may create a degree of turbulence in the system and so may slightly increase the discomfort however, we are only going to go at these things rather gently and as such neither of them should cause any major ongoing upset and should produce amelioration (improvement) of the condition going forward.

Now that we're turning our attention to tendon gliding (also referred to tendon elongation or tendon stretching... these terms are used interchangeably) I want to return to something I said earlier in the book about not doing a particular stretch of the affected finger. I am now going to row back a bit on this, in that tendon gliding is something which can be extremely useful but which, if applied incorrectly, inappropriately and unthinkingly, can cause substantial discomfort in trigger finger. To that end, I am going to show you three methods of gliding your tendons. We are going to start with the simplest and then we're going to do the slightly more complicated version and then end with the strongest and most complicated. I will explain why we are doing it in this order in a moment but for now, make sure that before you do any tendon gliding, that you have immersed your hand in the warm water first. Tendon gliding is best done when the hand and the forearm have been preheated in the way that I have described and ensure that they are done in the order that I advise.

These three methods are: The first is the standard stretch of the extrinsic finger flexors where we stretch both joints in the same direction at the same time. The second is when we stretch the FDS only and the third does FDS mainly but with greater tension caused by a fundamental change in the starting position of the stretch. First of all, let's take a look at the standard stretch that incorporates elongation (lengthening) of both of the extrinsic finger flexors.

The Standard Extrinsic Flexor Stretch (Stretch #1)

This is the stretch (Photo 9) that I mentioned in the early part of this book and is the one that I asked you not to do. The reason that we are doing this now is because it is the most intuitive and easiest of all stretches to do in the finger. The only problem with this stretch, is that under certain configurations of trigger finger, this might aggravate the symptoms. However, you won't know if this is true aggravation of the condition or if it is merely a response to being stretched. This is why I suggest that you continue with this stretch for one whole week and at the end of the week, when you fill in your diary, you may notice that pain levels are starting to creep up. If this happens, then you should drop this stretch and go on to the second stretch that I'm going to show you which is the isolated stretch for *flexor digitorum superficialis* (FDS).

Unfortunately, at the moment, it is difficult to predict whether this will cause any aggravation or not. By aggravation, I mean that the symptoms may become worse and by symptoms I mean the pain symptoms. It is unlikely that this will cause an increase in triggering although this is not beyond the bounds of possibility. Either way, a worsening of the symptoms will show up in the data over the seven-day diary. It is important when you do this stretch, that you are not overly aggressive. All you should feel is a gentle stretch which may be felt along the whole length of the finger and possibly into the wrist and even up into the forearm. Do not be concerned about this, however you should not stretch it to the point of provoking pain. There should be absolutely no tingling, pin and needles, numbness or sharp pain. The former three sensations mean that you are stretching a nerve and this is not advised.

This might appear odd that I suggest that 'sharp' pain should be avoided, because in the book on the ManTTr® Protocol[5], I advocate evoking pains which tend to be sharp in nature however, I only do this in relation to the application of the massage techniques on the muscles specifically and never during a stretch. If you feel a sharp sensation during a stretch, it usually means that you have gone beyond these soft tissues' natural elasticity and have evoked a situation whereby some of the soft tissue has been damaged. Obviously, this is to be avoided.

In terms of treatment frequency, this stretch should be done only after you have immersed your hand in warm water and done your exercises in the same. It must not be overdone and I would strongly advise not to do this unless you have bathed your hand in warm water for a <u>full 10 minutes</u>. While I have advised you to do the immersion in water and the associated exercise twice a day, you can do this immersion and stretch more than twice a day if you have the time and inclination... very few people do! Overall, if I were to be pushed on what I think the maximum amount of immersion in water and stretching would be, I would suggest it would be no more than four times a day.

Photo 9:Standard Stretch of Extrinsic Finger Flexors (Stretch #1)

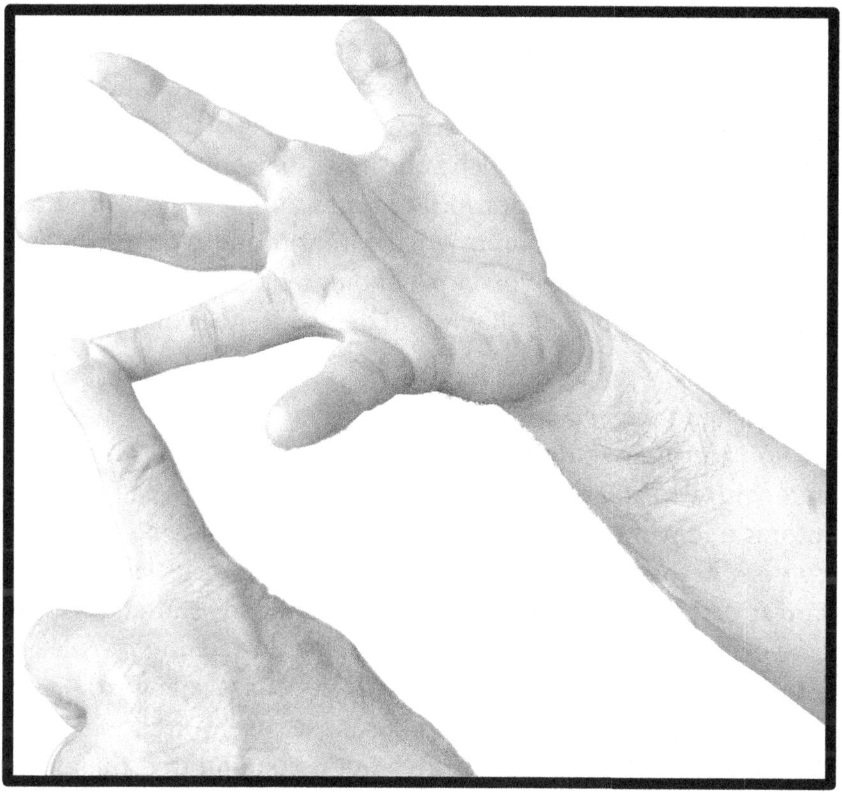

Reproduced with kind permission from the author and publisher of 'The Manual Therapy Trigger Finger (ManTTr®) Protocol[5]

Please bear in mind that by doubling the amount of exercise and immersion that you do, does not mean that you will half the rate at which your trigger finger improves. It is likely that the optimum amount of intervention will vary between individuals given that heating rates, flexibility and tissue pliability will vary. The more willing a tissue is to move, the more likely change will take place and conversely, the more resistant a body is to movement, the longer it will take for change to occur should any change occur at all. If this standard stretch is working for you, and by that,

I mean that if the symptoms are continuing to abate on your weekly measurements with reduction of pain and/or a reduction in your modified SST score, then you are doing the correct stretch for you. If this is the case, do not attempt the isolation stretch of FDS. This is only indicated if you have no change in your symptoms after the standard stretch or if your symptoms have worsened.

OK, so let's again take a look at where we are in our strategy for you treating our own trigger finger. Figure 7 provides the overview so far indicating that you should have completed three weeks of diary. You have either made or acquired a splint which you should be continuing to use to rest your finger at night and at appropriate times during the day. You are also doing immersion of your hand, wrist, forearm and elbow in warm water and while in the water you are bending and straightening your fingers at least 10 times, moving slowly and deliberately, avoiding pain as much as possible.

You are now going to engage with an initial stretch which is the standard stretch and you are going to do this for a week and during that week, you will continue with your diary. For this intervention, you will pay heed to your symptoms and whether or not they are improving, staying the same or getting worse. At the end of week three, you will need to decide whether the standard stretch is working or not. As we have already stated, this will, or should, be evident by the scores that you have recorded during Week 3. Normally, the key change will be in 'pain' which usually manifests as an increased ache in the palm of the hand. If this is the case, you should STOP stretch #1 and move on to the next stretch but if you find that things are improving after stretch#1 you should continue with this stretch and skip any other stretches. This means that your next step is to go on to auto-massage (self-administered massage) of your affected side's forearm in Chapter 6.

However, if, after stretch #1 your symptoms are either staying the same or getting worse, you should drop this standard stretch (stretch #1) and add another week of stretch for the FDS which is the first isolation stretch or stretch #2. Still, first things first! Before you make any decisions about which stretch is best (if any) you need to give stretch #1 a chance, so next, fill out the daily diaries for stretch #1.

Figure 7: Summary of Progress to Week 3

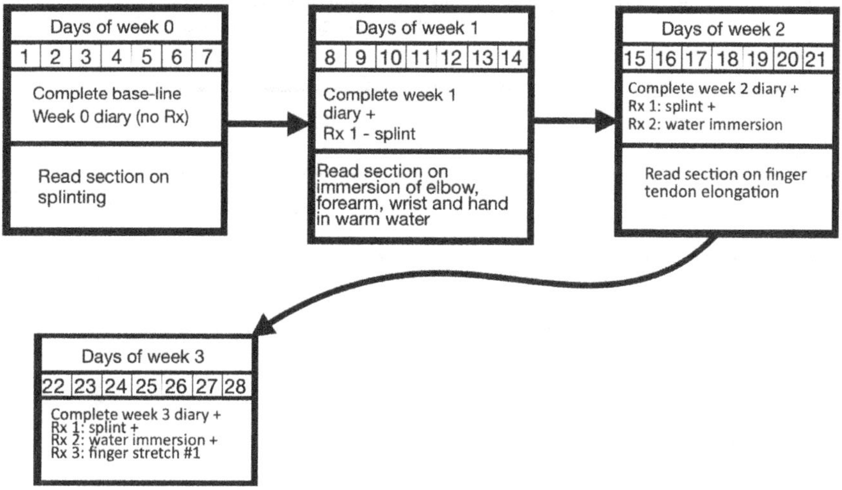

Week 3 Diaries

Modified SST (stages of stenosing tenosynovitis) Score Key:
0 Normal finger movement
1 Uneven finger movement (looks smooth but feels rough)
2 Triggering or clicking or catching (looks a bit jerky, not fully smooth)
3 Finger locking in a bent or straight position but can unlock by active finger movements
4 Finger locking in a bent or straight position but unlocked by passive finger movements
5 Locked finger in bent or straightened position but cannot be unlocked at all
Pain Numeric Rating Scale (PNRS) Key:
No pain 0 1 2 3 4 5 6 7 8 9 10 Worst pain Imaginable

Trigger Finger Daily Diary		Week 3 Day 1	
Date:		Modified SST score (see Key) 0-5	Pain Level (PNRS) (see key) 0-10
On waking after main sleep	At rest		
	On bending/straightening		
During most active period	At rest		
	On bending/straightening		
Just prior to main sleep	At rest		
	On bending/straightening		
My trigger finger today has:		Yes	No
	Disturbed my sleep		
	Prevented me from doing an activity I wanted or needed to do		
STATE AND DESCRIBE ACTIVITY:			
Medication for Trigger Finger: Frequency.....................times/day Medication Name: Total daily dose:		Yes	No
	Can you make a full fist just before my main sleep?		
	Can you straighten your fingers fully just before my main sleep?		

Trigger Finger Daily Diary		Week 3 Day 2	
Date:		Modified SST score (see Key) 0-5	Pain Level (PNRS) (see key) 0-10
On waking after main sleep	At rest		
	On bending/straightening		
During most active period	At rest		
	On bending/straightening		
Just prior to main sleep	At rest		
	On bending/straightening		
My trigger finger today has:		Yes	No
	Disturbed my sleep		
	Prevented me from doing an activity I wanted or needed to do		
STATE AND DESCRIBE ACTIVITY:			
Medication for Trigger Finger: Frequency.....................times/day Medication Name: Total daily dose:		Yes	No
	Can you make a full fist just before my main sleep?		
	Can you straighten your fingers fully just before my main sleep?		

Trigger Finger Daily Diary		Week 3 Day 3	
Date:		Modified SST score (see Key) 0-5	Pain Level (PNRS) (see key) 0-10
On waking after main sleep	At rest		
	On bending/straightening		
During most active period	At rest		
	On bending/straightening		
Just prior to main sleep	At rest		
	On bending/straightening		

My trigger finger today has:	Yes	No
Disturbed my sleep		
Prevented me from doing an activity I wanted or needed to do		
STATE AND DESCRIBE ACTIVITY:		

Medication for Trigger Finger: Frequency..................times/day Medication Name: Total daily dose:	Yes	No
Can you make a full fist just before my main sleep?		
Can you straighten your fingers fully just before my main sleep?		

Trigger Finger Daily Diary		Week 3 Day 4	
Date:		Modified SST score (see Key) 0-5	Pain Level (PNRS) (see key) 0-10
On waking after main sleep	At rest		
	On bending/straightening		
During most active period	At rest		
	On bending/straightening		
Just prior to main sleep	At rest		
	On bending/straightening		

My trigger finger today has:	Yes	No
Disturbed my sleep		
Prevented me from doing an activity I wanted or needed to do		
STATE AND DESCRIBE ACTIVITY:		

Medication for Trigger Finger: Frequency..................times/day Medication Name: Total daily dose:	Yes	No
Can you make a full fist just before my main sleep?		
Can you straighten your fingers fully just before my main sleep?		

Trigger Finger Daily Diary		Week 3 Day 5	
Date:		Modified SST score (see Key) 0-5	Pain Level (PNRS) (see key) 0-10
On waking after main sleep	At rest		
	On bending/straightening		
During most active period	At rest		
	On bending/straightening		
Just prior to main sleep	At rest		
	On bending/straightening		

My trigger finger today has:	Yes	No
Disturbed my sleep		
Prevented me from doing an activity I wanted or needed to do		
STATE AND DESCRIBE ACTIVITY:		
Medication for Trigger Finger: Frequency...................times/day Medication Name: Total daily dose:	Yes	No
Can you make a full fist just before my main sleep?		
Can you straighten your fingers fully just before my main sleep?		

Trigger Finger Daily Diary		Week 3 Day 6	
Date:		Modified SST score (see Key) 0-5	Pain Level (PNRS) (see key) 0-10
On waking after main sleep	At rest		
	On bending/straightening		
During most active period	At rest		
	On bending/straightening		
Just prior to main sleep	At rest		
	On bending/straightening		

My trigger finger today has:	Yes	No
Disturbed my sleep		
Prevented me from doing an activity I wanted or needed to do		
STATE AND DESCRIBE ACTIVITY:		
Medication for Trigger Finger: Frequency...................times/day Medication Name: Total daily dose:	Yes	No
Can you make a full fist just before my main sleep?		
Can you straighten your fingers fully just before my main sleep?		

Trigger Finger Daily Diary		Week 3 Day 7	
Date:		Modified SST score (see Key) 0-5	Pain Level (PNRS) (see key) 0-10
On waking after main sleep	At rest		
	On bending/straightening		
During most active period	At rest		
	On bending/straightening		
Just prior to main sleep	At rest		
	On bending/straightening		

My trigger finger today has:	Yes	No
Disturbed my sleep		
Prevented me from doing an activity I wanted or needed to do		
STATE AND DESCRIBE ACTIVITY:		
Medication for Trigger Finger: Frequency...................times/day Medication Name: Total daily dose:	Yes	No
Can you make a full fist just before my main sleep?		
Can you straighten your fingers fully just before my main sleep?		

Isolation Stretch for FDS (stretch #2)

If stretch #1 fails causing either symptom worsening or no change (statis) we are going to drop stretch #1 and do the 2nd tendon glide (stretch #2). This can potentially mix up the weeks that we have, so far, named chronologically from Week 0 through Week 3. Although we are now, technically, in Week 4, in reality, what we are really doing, is repeating Week 3 (stretch/elongation). However, we need to keep counting the days that we have been undertaking this self-treatment regimen. As such, we need to deviate slightly from our standard numbering. So, as long as we are in a “tendon gliding phase” we will refer to this as a ‘repeat Week 3’. The isolation stretch for FDS, that we are about to do (stretch #2) will be referred to specifically as ‘repeat Week 3i’. If we should go on to stretch #3, this will be called ‘repeat of Week 3ii’. This is why, from here, to the final treatment, the reader will need to enter the days relating to whichever week they are on which is going to be in theory, Week 4 (called repeat week 3i) but could in fact, if there are two repeated weeks of Week 3, we could be going up to week 5 (called repeat week 3ii). Confused? I hope not! Anyway, with that said, let's now take a look at the first of our repeats of Week 3 sessions which is the isolation stretch for FDS (stretch 2; repeat Week 3i).

The purpose of this stretch (Photo 10) is to attempt to lengthen the FDS but to limit the stretch to the FDP. In doing this, we are trying to slide FDS over FDP because the latter will remain relatively still in relation to the former during the stretch. This idea of creating separation is to allow the muscles to re-establish their natural rhythm of contraction as, in the theory that we are currently applying, we make the presumption that this rhythm between these muscles has been interrupted. Now I know you might be getting a bit bored with me saying this, but I do go into a lot more detail in my book on the ManTTr® Protocol[5]. The self-treatment that I am describing to you in this book that you are reading, is partly based on the theory that underpins the ManTTr® Protocol[5] intervention and also, in the "ManTTr®" book, I try to explain what I think is the overall cause of trigger finger. This causation theory is novel and is the first serious attempt to bring all of the strands that appear to operate in producing what is, otherwise, a condition of unknown origin. However, for the purposes of this self-help guide, I will merely describe the isolation stretch for FDS.

In the photograph below (Photo 10) you can see that the stretch of the FDS is much more complicated than the standard stretch for the extrinsic finger flexors. It may take a little bit of time and effort to work out how to best position the fingers of your opposite hand but, just follow the photograph and you will get there eventually! The idea here, is to prevent, or minimise, the stretch of FDP by flexing the tip of the affected finger. This loosens FDP while, at the same time, we try to bend the joint associated with FDS slightly backwards. Again, we do not want to apply excessive pressure to this. You may feel a mild pull around the base of the affected finger in the palm or even in the wrist but rarely in the forearm, although this is possible. In terms of frequency, this will be the same as the standard stretch and it is also true to say that this should only be done after the immersion in water. At the end of a week of stretching, using this isolated stretch (stretch #2) the increased ache caused by stretch #1 should be reducing. If it is not, STOP ALL STRETCHES but continue with the immersion and the splint. Once the pain has returned to 'your' normal (as measured by diary entries) resume stretch #2. Additional diaries for 'repeat Week 4' (tendon gliding) are in Appendix 2.

Photo 10: Isolated Stretch for FDS (Stretch #2)

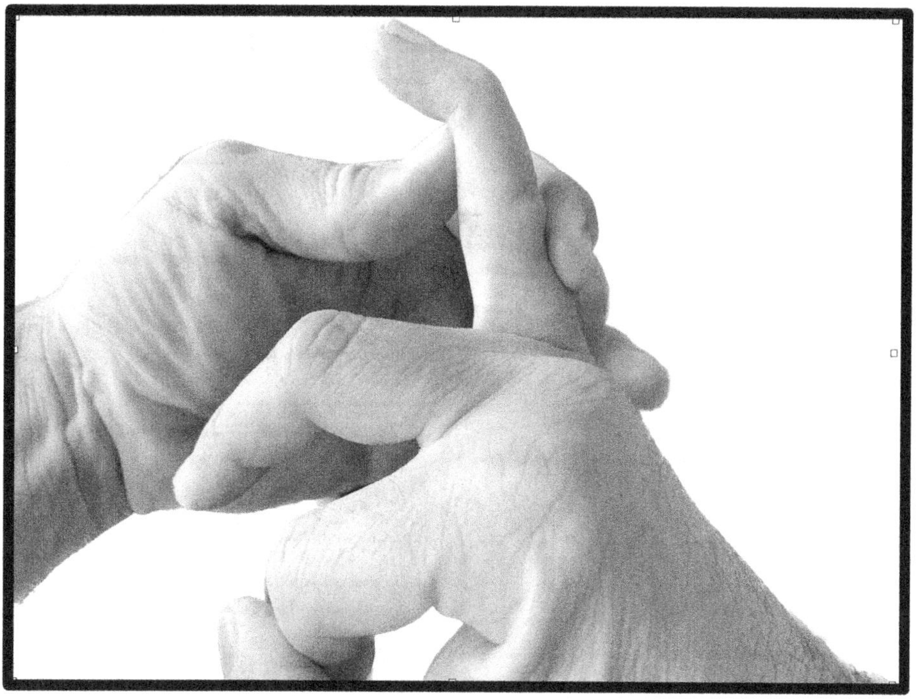

Reproduced with kind permission from the author and publisher of 'The Manual Therapy Trigger Finger (ManTTr®) Protocol[5]

If you would like to see a video of stretch #2, click on the link:

https://www.youtube.com/watch?v=zO-zYASnbqQ

So now, let's take a look at where we are in terms of the overall approach to self-treatment. Figure 8 shows the progress for repeat Week 3i. During the completion of this treatment and the associated diary entries, it could be timely to look back over your progress (or lack of) and perhaps jot a few things down in relation to this process and maybe send me a short email (given at the back of this book) to let me know how things are going. It would be great to hear from you either way!

Figure 8: Summary of Progress to Repeat Week 3i

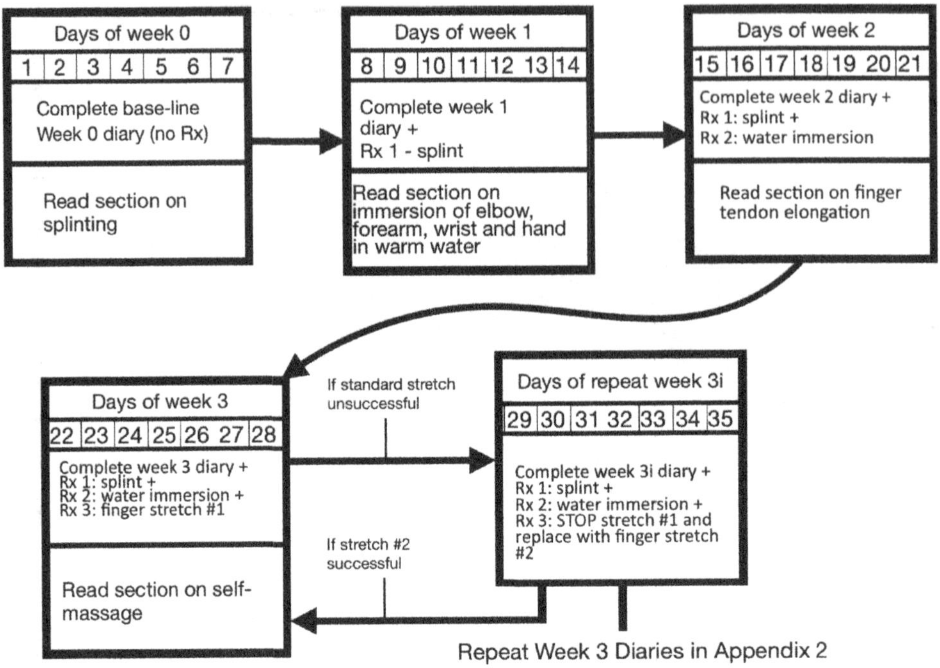

<u>Tendon Glide in Wrist Extension (Stretch #3)</u>

This final stretch that I want to show you for the affected finger is the strongest of all the stretches and is primarily for FDS. This should never be done as a first stretch and should only be done if you are able to complete the first two. If the stretch #2 causes pain then you <u>should not</u> do stretch #3 as it is likely to cause even more discomfort. However, if you find that stretch #2 has neither improved nor worsened the problem, then you can progress to stretch #3. However, because of the extreme position of this stretch, you should not do this if you have problems with your wrist. Even if your wrist is okay, this stretch needs to be done gently, progressively and carefully. The process for conducting this stretch is as follows: Firstly, place your hand flat on a work surface and then roll your weight over it so that the wrist bends backwards (see Photo 11a). You do not need to force this so make sure that this is not painful. If it is painful, then you should not do this stretch and should consult a health professional as this movement should not be painful even when over-pressure is applied. Secondly, you should try to get your index finger of your opposite hand underneath you're affected finger, between the two knuckles of the affected finger on the affected hand without having to lift your palm off the surface (see Photo 11b).

Photo 11: a through f Wrist Extension Finger Stretch (Stretch #3)

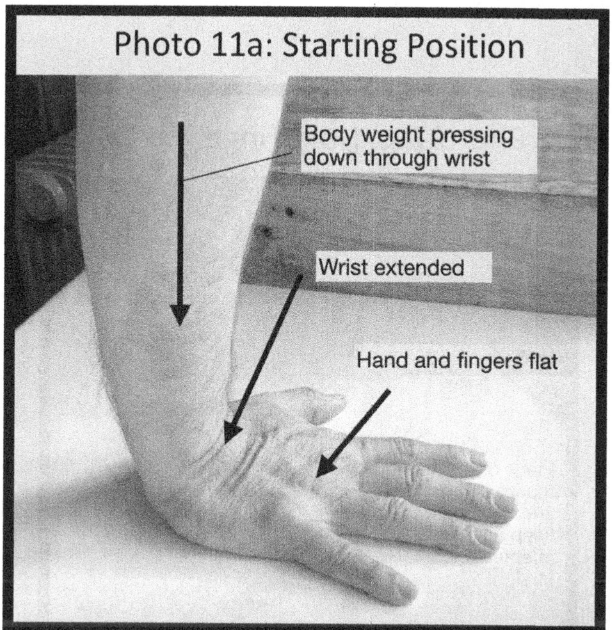

Photo 11a: Starting Position

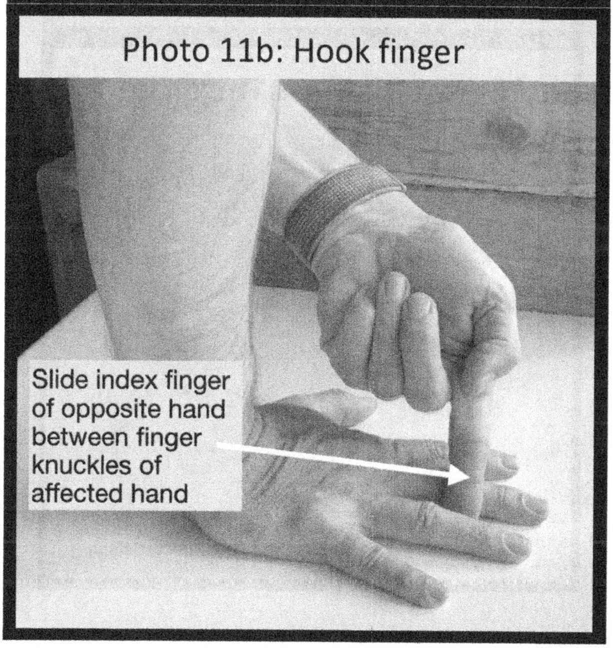

Photo 11b: Hook finger

Then you stretch this by placing your opposite (usually index) finger under your affected finger (see photo 11c). Hold it there and at the same time, place your opposite thumb over the first knuckle on the affected finger to bend it slightly backwards and hold this position for around 30 seconds or less, but certainly no more

Photo 11c: Hold Finger

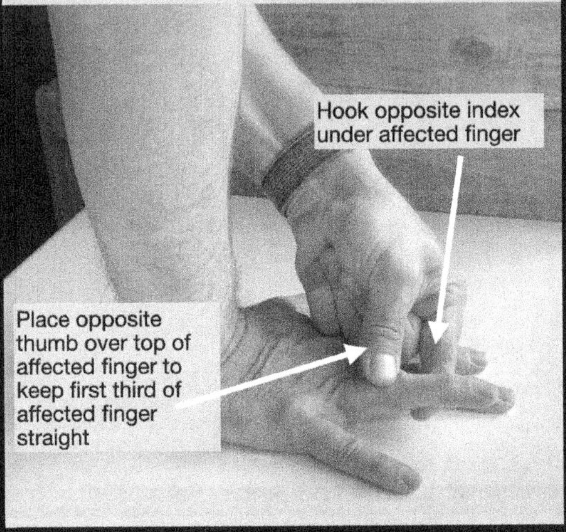

Photo 11d: Move Fingertip

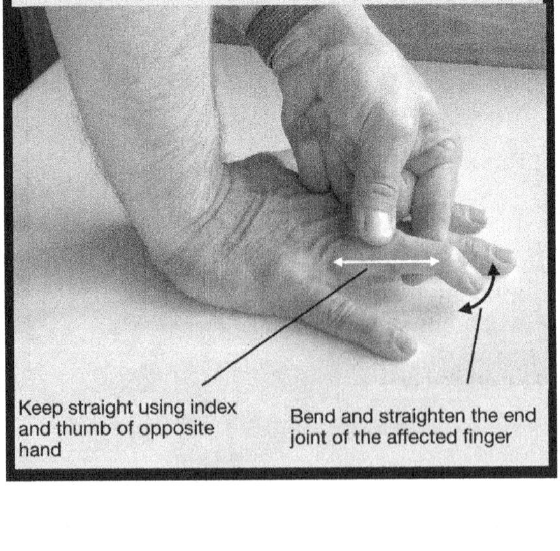

If you would like to see a video of stretch #3, click on the link:

https://www.youtube.com/watch?v=B5BVPhke7Kc

Photo 11e: Palm Discomfort During Stretch

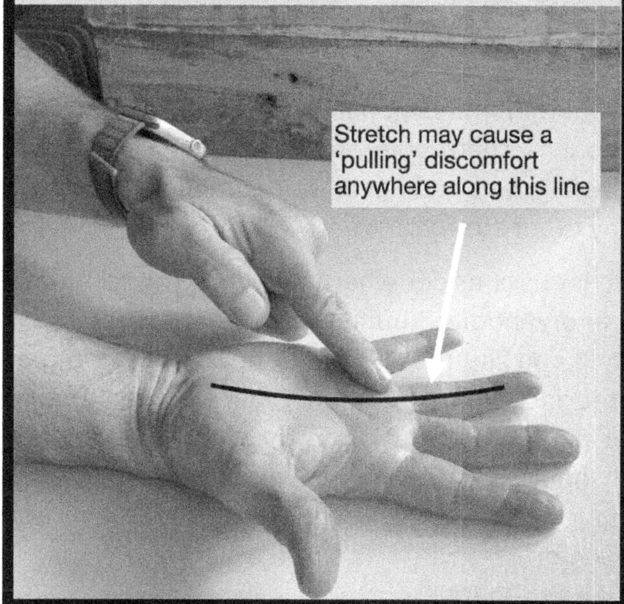

Photo 11f: Forearm Discomfort During Stretch

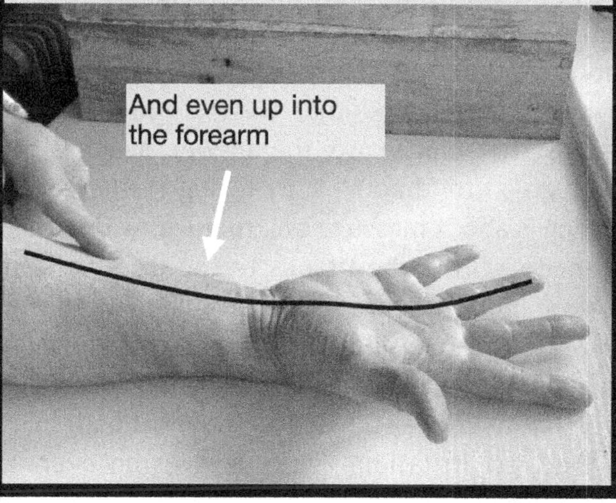

There may, however, just be the feeling of a stretch but if pain appears or increases, stop the stretch. Otherwise, after holding for 30 seconds or less, try to make the fingertip of your affected finger bend and straighten (see Photo 11d). After this, there can be a residual sense of discomfort which is really just the after-effect of the stretch and this can be felt either just in the palm (Photo 11e) or in the palm and the forearm (Photo 11f). This is usually short lived but if it persists beyond a few minutes, it can be relieved by conducting another immersion in warm water as previously instructed. At no point should a sharp pain be evoked. Equally, there should be no sensation of tingling, pins and needles or numbness experienced during or after this or any other stretch.

So, once again, let us consider where we are in the scheme of things with regard to our interventions. You may also want to look back at your data to see if that tells you anything. Figure 9 shows a rather more complicated picture with the inclusion of tendon glide #3. The complexity is partly brought about by the interruption in the flow of numbering but also in terms of what should be done in the event that none of the stretches are effective in changing your trigger finger status and even may have caused increased discomfort.

There may be two likely possibilities for this: the first is that the repeated stretch and variation of the stretch may have created some degree of irritation of the tissues in which case, the next stage is to stop all stretches and let this settle and while this is occurring, move on to Chapter 6. The other possibility is that there is potential tethering between the structures that need to be mobilised and that this tethering has not yet being sufficiently mobilised in which case, the answer, again, is to abandon the stretching and to go on to Chapter 6. By taking the next step and moving to Chapter 6 which is about massage of structures within the forearm, this may be sufficient to agitate the tissues to the extent that they become freer and therefore more prepared to be stretched. In this event, you will need to return to the stretch. Which of these stretches that you return to, is a matter for you to decide and my advice would be that you would choose the stretch that you feel gives you the most benefit or looking at it another way, the least irritation. Figure 8 gives an overall summary of where we are at the moment in terms of our intervention for self-assistance.

Figure 9: Summary of Progress to Repeat Week ii

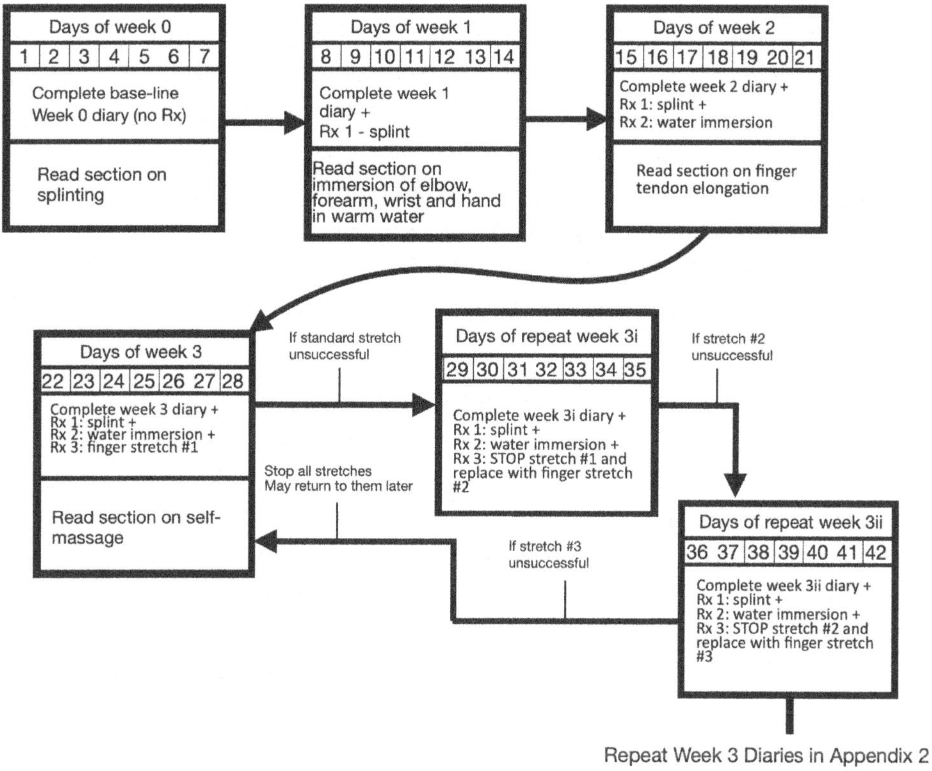

It would be great if this process could be dynamic so to this end, I would welcome your correspondence, particularly if you are uncertain about anything that I am saying or even if you would like to tell me about your experiences for good or not so good! There is no method of intervention that guarantees success and that's actually a good thing because it means that there is always room for improvement!

Chapter 6: Week 4, 4th Treatment: Self-Massage

I'm sure you will remember that at the beginning of this book, I told you not to massage your palm. If you look on the internet you will see this advice given pretty much everywhere but, in my opinion, this is not the thing to do. The reason why this is not the thing to do is because the problem of trigger finger does not arise from the hand but from the forearm[5]. In fact, it's not anywhere in the forearm, it is a specific place in the forearm that you have to find. I say this is a specific place, but it is a specific place which isn't always the same place for everyone, and that's why you have to find it.

In this section I am going to show you, not only how to find the specific area that you need to massage but, how to massage it and how long to massage it for. I will also tell you the frequency with which you need to massage. Unlike all the other treatments that I have advised in this self-help book, this is the one that you **NEVER** do every day. In fact, there are a series of rules that you need to apply when doing this massage. It is something that can be easily overdone and in so doing, it is quite conceivable that not only will you make the problem in your hand worse, but also, you will create new problems in the forearm.

The reason that we massage where we do, is to try to create a degree of mobility in the area which, in turn, does a number of things. Firstly, it inputs mechanical energy into an area of the body which, I believe, has become depleted and immobile. Secondly, we are trying to increase the local blood supply so that any mechanical effects that we have in this area, such as micro-soft tissue disturbance, will quickly heal. Thirdly, we are trying to change the biomechanics of the muscles in that we are attempting to correct the angle of pull exerted on the tendons in the hand which are those same tendons that give rise to the symptoms of trigger finger.

Of course, this treatment in isolation is unlikely to succeed. This is why I have given you three distinct things to do prior to getting to this point. First of all, we've applied the splint to try and allow any inflammation, regardless of where it may be, to settle as much as is practicably possible and then we have done some exercise in warm water to make sure that the tissues are fully mobile and pliable and then we have applied one or more stretches. Of these stretches, you need to decide which is the most beneficial for you and then stick only to that one. So now, we're going into another series of interventions which will capitalise on all the groundwork that we have done over the previous weeks. On no account whatsoever should you do this massage unless you have completed the whole series of interventions that I've advised prior to this. If you do, you will almost certainly create more problems… so don't do it!

Now before we begin with our self (sometimes called auto-) massage, you need to make sure that your thumb on your opposite hand is prepared. To prepare your thumb (that will be doing the massaging) you need to have your nail short and your hands washed thoroughly. Make sure that your short thumb nail is filed smooth. This is to ensure that you do not damage your skin by having nails which are too long. This is particularly important for people who have diabetes (even if the blood sugars are well controlled and stable) as breaching the skin poses distinct dangers as, should a skin breach (cut, wound) become infected, it can lead to very serious consequences including limb loss. Having prepared your thumb, we now need to consider how you begin the self-massage. Make sure you follow these instructions carefully and do not deviate or make it up as you go along!

Now we are ready to start with the self-massage. You can do this in any position you wish but most people prefer to be seated. Once positioned, we need to find the area to treat. Firstly, we activate the affected muscle in the forearm by pressing the tip of the affected finger up against the tip of the thumb on the same hand. This movement is known as "opposition". Just as a matter of interest, the action of "opposition" of the thumb is something that is unique to humans. If you look at the palm with relaxed fingers in a neutral position (either actively bent or straightened) you will see that the thumb is orientated at 90^0 to the palm (see Photo 12a). This means that the thumb is able to move across the palm (see Photo 12b) but it is also able to move in the same direction as the fingers. One of the variants of trigger finger, is called trigger thumb. This is very common and tends to be more debilitating than trigger finger because there are many skilled actions that our hands perform that involve the thumb, especially those requiring precision. Just to remind you, that this book does not cover trigger thumb as there are other ways of dealing with this because the thumb is a much more complex entity than the average finger and so a different approach has to be taken.

Photo 12: a and b Thumb 'Neutral' Position and Opposition

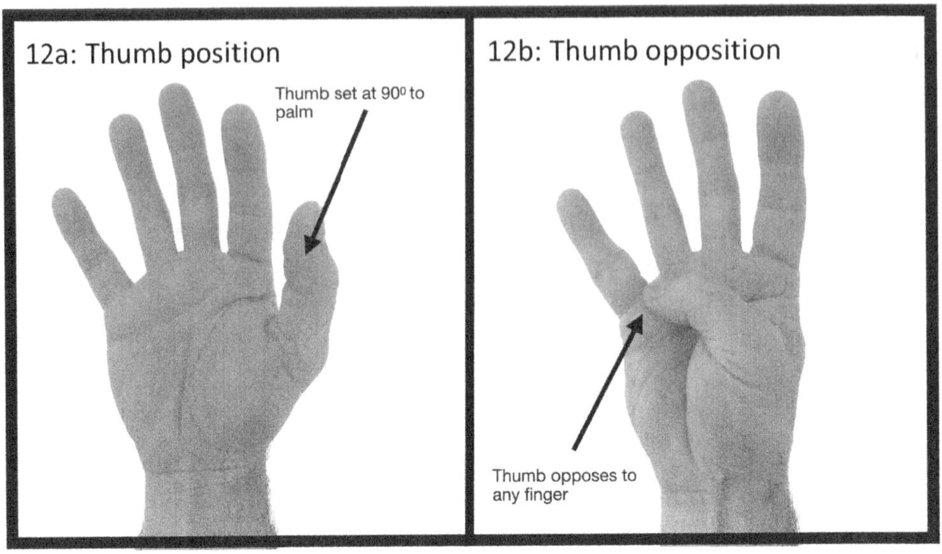

Photo 13: Opposition, Palpation & Massage of Affected Area of Forearm

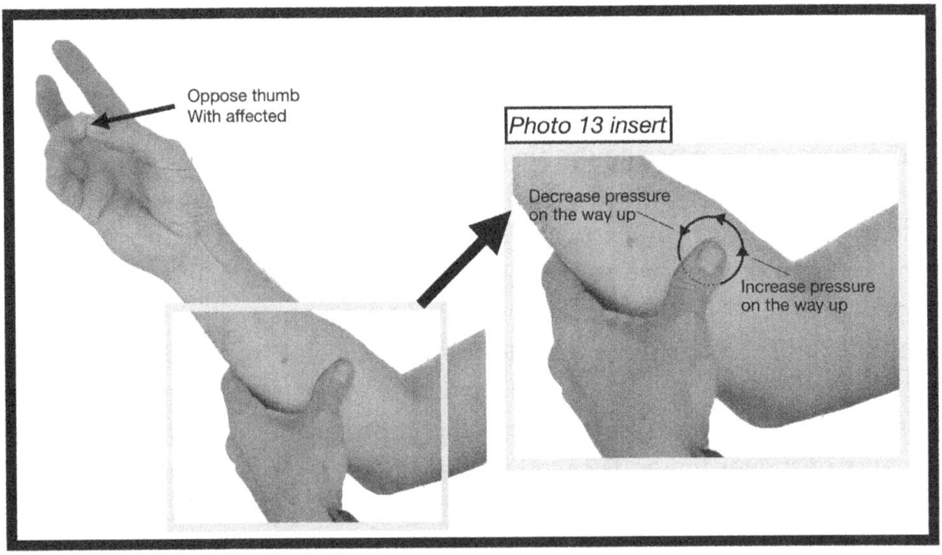

So, let's get back to our auto-mobilisation of our trigger finger and specifically, the identification of the target area: Having opposed the affected finger and the thumb, we can now use the thumb of the opposite hand to feel up the forearm, along the line of contracting muscle of the affected (opposed) finger (Photo 13). By doing this, you are looking for a 'raised' tender area in the forearm. To do this effectively, do the following: maintaining the affected finger and thumb in opposition, slide your opposite thumb up and down the forearm. As you move up and down the forearm, use the thumb pad (see Photo 14a) not the tip (see Photo 14b) making sure you are applying pressure into the tensed muscle and that you are moving slowly. You are looking for a tender and/or raised or thickened area which is also part of the muscle that is being contracted. It can take quite a bit of finding but with sufficient pressure and patience, you will feel an area that is more tender than the surrounding area. Once you think you have found this, you then change the position of your thumb so that you are pressing the tip of your thumb (see of Photo 14b) into the area that you feel you have identified.

Photo 14: a and b Thumb Pad and Thumb Tip

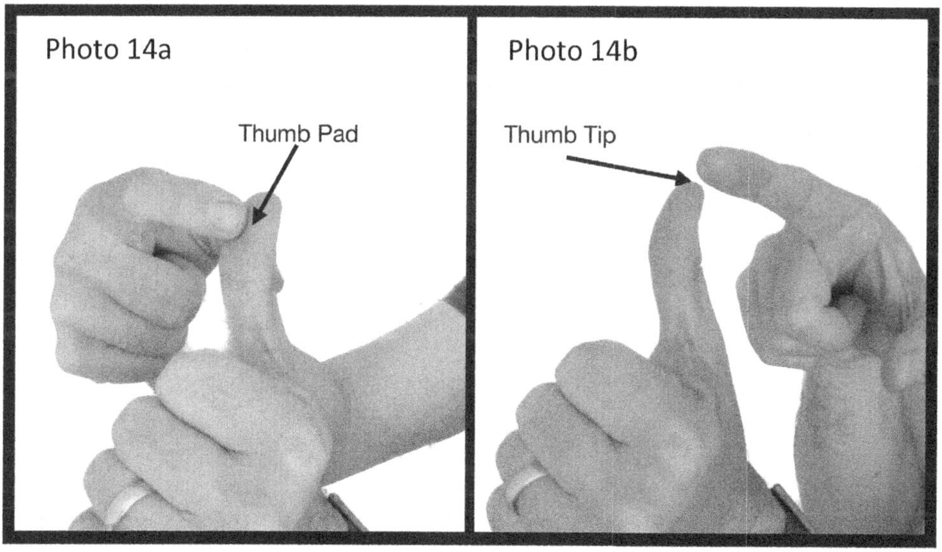

Making sure that you are still opposing your affected finger and your thumb as shown in Photo 13, press into the sensitive area using the tip of your opposite thumb and agitate it up and down. This should increase the tenderness and may even produce a sense of sharpness. Then, stop the agitation but maintain your finger over the sensitive area and now, still holding the pressure into your forearm with your opposite thumb and relax the opposition of your from and affected finger. Once you do this, you should feel the soreness or tenderness in the forearm disappear. You do not need to press any harder than you are pressing so make sure you maintain this level of pressure for the rest of the massage. You then re-oppose the affected finger and the thumb and maintaining the pressure with your opposite thumb on your forearm and you should notice that the discomfort comes back. If this happens, it means you have found the area that needs to be massaged.

To massage this, you return to applying your **thumb pad** (Photo 14a) over the area, reapply the pressure and then massage in circles (left thumb on right forearm = anti-(counter) clockwise; right thumb on left forearm = clockwise) with the thumb in what is often called thumb needing (see insert on Photo 13). This should have a slight variation in pressure whereby when you are pushing your thumb up, in the direction of your radius (the forearm bone on the side of the thumb), you should press slightly heavier and then gradually, just ease off as you move round to the bottom of the massage circle, and then press in again as you rise up over the tender area. You should do this for 20 slow circles, making sure that you stay over the sensitive area. If you find that this is becoming increasingly painful, you can do fewer circles and/or ease off the pressure on your thumb pad but maintain the circular massage over the area.

If you would like to see a video of me conducting the forearm massage, go to the following link:

https://www.youtube.com/watch?v=agVkwEa1b6s

Once you have completed your 20 rotations of the auto massage, remove your hand and relax the affected hand and use your opposite hand to rub over the area that you've just massaged. It is not unusual for this area to be reddened. This should fade fairly quickly but in some cases, you may notice that a bruise forms. This in and of itself is not a problem however, just as a matter of precaution, you should never massage once a bruise has formed. You must wait until the bruise has COMPLETELY DISAPPEARED before you restart massaging it again.

As mentioned earlier, you must never massage every day. The earliest you should re-massage this area, is after four days from the previous massage. Do not be tempted to fiddle or prod or poke this area as it will merely prolong tenderness. Remember, that if my theory is right about the cause of trigger finger, the area that you've just been massaging, is the area that is causing the trigger finger. This is essentially a biomechanical problem. If you massage over an area that is either injured, or dysfunctional or whatever, it is more likely to bruise than if it was not injured. It is also more likely to be tender than if it hadn't been injured and therefore it requires more time to settle. Do not ignore this advice! It is absolutely essential for this approach to be successful that you have patience and that you give it time to make whatever changes it needs to make in relation and in response to the massage that you have given. In essence, your tissues need to recalibrate themselves to the new normal and this can take time. Even after you have completed the whole cycle that I recommend (a cycle of four mobilisations; see item 6 of the massage schedule below) you need to give the tissues additional time to allow this recalibration or remodelling to take place and this can take between three and six months.

You may feel that you haven't done much, and you may not have but given the tissue's relative frailty, and underlying dysfunction, do not be surprised if this bruises and or feels tender. Do not underestimate the effect that this very focused massage will have on your tissues. This is why I do not recommend that you do this if you have any problems with your skin or you have inflammatory conditions such as rheumatoid arthritis or you have congenital problems such as amyloidosis, haemophilia, or vascular or sensation distorting or reducing neurological dysfunction. However, it is important that you continue with the stretching and the warm water immersion but, after having completed two massages (no less than four days apart) you may then stop using the splint but now is the time to restart the stretching if you have postponed it as discussed earlier in the book. This is because we now want to push mobility to make the tissues move from here on in, unless there is a spike in pain for some reason, in which case, the splint may be used when resting the hand. Otherwise, movement, at this stage in self-treatment, is a priority!

The Massage Schedule

1. Once you have settled on a particular stretch and there is a sign of either progression or no progress, and that you have completed at least one whole week of your preferred stretch, you may then start the massage stage.
2. Follow the guidance on massage (Chapter 6); do not cut corners.
3. Once you have found the part of the forearm that is most likely to be the target area, you may commence the mobilisation but only mobilise this area and no other even if there are other tender locations in the forearm unconnected with the triggering finger.
4. Having found the location, massage with moderate pressure for about 20 circular movements or do as many as you can up to that number and/or ease the pressure.
5. Refrain from doing any further massage if the area bruises. If there is a bruise you must not massage over that area (or even in its vicinity) anymore until the bruise has **completely** gone. Do not be tempted to massage over this area if there remains even the slightest discoloration of the skin.
6. Notwithstanding the caveat in #5 above, you may massage the area again four days after the previous massage. For example, if you massage on Monday you may massage again (as long as there is no bruising) on Thursday. After your second mobilisation, you may massage again in a further four days. After your third massage, you may massage for a 4th and final time four days later.
7. After your 4th massage, you must now stop the massages but continue with the stretches and the water treatment. Extra diaries for continued massage can be found in Appendix 3.
8. Completing #7 above may take six weeks, depending on bruising. Once the cycle of 4 massages is complete, stop this but continue the water treatment and stretches for a further six-weeks. Use your hand normally throughout this time. If, six-weeks after stopping the massage, there is noticeable improvement (qualitative or quantitatively) repeat another cycle of 4 massages. If there is no change in your condition, then you need to go on to the next stage of treatment. However, it must be stated that any further treatment will not be self-administered but will require the intervention of a health professional or body worker.

Modified SST (stages of stenosing tenosynovitis) Score Key:
0 Normal finger movement
1 Uneven finger movement (looks smooth but feels rough)
2 Triggering or clicking or catching (looks a bit jerky, not fully smooth)
3 Finger locking in a bent or straight position but can unlock by active finger movements
4 Finger locking in a bent or straight position but unlocked by passive finger movements
5 Locked finger in bent or straightened position but cannot be unlocked at all

Pain Numeric Rating Scale (PNRS) Key:

No pain											Worst pain Imaginable
	0	1	2	3	4	5	6	7	8	9	10

Trigger Finger Daily Diary		Week 4 Day 1	
Date:		Modified SST score (see Key) 0-5	Pain Level (PNRS) (see key) 0-10
On waking after main sleep	At rest		
	On bending/straightening		
During most active period	At rest		
	On bending/straightening		
Just prior to main sleep	At rest		
	On bending/straightening		

My trigger finger today has:	Yes	No
Disturbed my sleep		
Prevented me from doing an activity I wanted or needed to do STATE AND DESCRIBE ACTIVITY:		

Medication for Trigger Finger: Frequency……………….times/day Medication Name: Total daily dose:	Yes	No
Can you make a full fist just before my main sleep?		
Can you straighten your fingers fully just before my main sleep?		

Trigger Finger Daily Diary		Week 4 Day 3	
Date:		Modified SST score (see Key) 0-5	Pain Level (PNRS) (see key) 0-10
On waking after main sleep	At rest		
	On bending/straightening		
During most active period	At rest		
	On bending/straightening		
Just prior to main sleep	At rest		
	On bending/straightening		

My trigger finger today has:	Yes	No
Disturbed my sleep		
Prevented me from doing an activity I wanted or needed to do STATE AND DESCRIBE ACTIVITY:		

Medication for Trigger Finger: Frequency....................times/day Medication Name: Total daily dose:	Yes	No
Can you make a full fist just before my main sleep?		
Can you straighten your fingers fully just before my main sleep?		

Trigger Finger Daily Diary		Week 4 Day 2	
Date:		Modified SST score (see Key) 0-5	Pain Level (PNRS) (see key) 0-10
On waking after main sleep	At rest		
	On bending/straightening		
During most active period	At rest		
	On bending/straightening		
Just prior to main sleep	At rest		
	On bending/straightening		

My trigger finger today has:	Yes	No
Disturbed my sleep		
Prevented me from doing an activity I wanted or needed to do STATE AND DESCRIBE ACTIVITY:		

Medication for Trigger Finger: Frequency....................times/day Medication Name: Total daily dose:	Yes	No
Can you make a full fist just before my main sleep?		
Can you straighten your fingers fully just before my main sleep?		

Trigger Finger Daily Diary		Week 4 Day 4	
Date:		Modified SST score (see Key) 0-5	Pain Level (PNRS) (see key) 0-10
On waking after main sleep	At rest		
	On bending/straightening		
During most active period	At rest		
	On bending/straightening		
Just prior to main sleep	At rest		
	On bending/straightening		

My trigger finger today has:	Yes	No
Disturbed my sleep		
Prevented me from doing an activity I wanted or needed to do		
STATE AND DESCRIBE ACTIVITY:		
Medication for Trigger Finger: Frequency.………………..times/day Medication Name: Total daily dose:	Yes	No
Can you make a full fist just before my main sleep?		
Can you straighten your fingers fully just before my main sleep?		

Trigger Finger Daily Diary		Week 4 Day 5	
Date:		Modified SST score (see Key) 0-5	Pain Level (PNRS) (see key) 0-10
On waking after main sleep	At rest		
	On bending/straightening		
During most active period	At rest		
	On bending/straightening		
Just prior to main sleep	At rest		
	On bending/straightening		

My trigger finger today has:	Yes	No
Disturbed my sleep		
Prevented me from doing an activity I wanted or needed to do		
STATE AND DESCRIBE ACTIVITY:		
Medication for Trigger Finger: Frequency.………………..times/day Medication Name: Total daily dose:	Yes	No
Can you make a full fist just before my main sleep?		
Can you straighten your fingers fully just before my main sleep?		

Trigger Finger Daily Diary		Week 4 Day 6	
Date:		Modified SST score (see Key) 0-5	Pain Level (PNRS) (see key) 0-10
On waking after main sleep	At rest		
	On bending/straightening		
During most active period	At rest		
	On bending/straightening		
Just prior to main sleep	At rest		
	On bending/straightening		

My trigger finger today has:	Yes	No
Disturbed my sleep		
Prevented me from doing an activity I wanted or needed to do		
STATE AND DESCRIBE ACTIVITY:		
Medication for Trigger Finger: Frequency.....................times/day Medication Name: Total daily dose:	Yes	No
Can you make a full fist just before my main sleep?		
Can you straighten your fingers fully just before my main sleep?		

Trigger Finger Daily Diary		Week 4 Day 7	
Date:		Modified SST score (see Key) 0-5	Pain Level (PNRS) (see key) 0-10
On waking after main sleep	At rest		
	On bending/straightening		
During most active period	At rest		
	On bending/straightening		
Just prior to main sleep	At rest		
	On bending/straightening		

My trigger finger today has:	Yes	No
Disturbed my sleep		
Prevented me from doing an activity I wanted or needed to do		
STATE AND DESCRIBE ACTIVITY:		
Medication for Trigger Finger: Frequency.....................times/day Medication Name: Total daily dose:	Yes	No
Can you make a full fist just before my main sleep?		
Can you straighten your fingers fully just before my main sleep?		

Chapter 7: Has the Self-Treatment Worked?

On one level, you will know instinctively whether your trigger finger has improved or not, but sometimes there is doubt over whether improvement has occurred because the memory of our past problems tends to be very short and unreliable. This is why I have asked you to make a daily record of the state of your trigger finger both in terms of the quality of movement and the pain. I've also asked you to make a note of a particular function that you find difficult. It is on the basis of these three recorded metrics (pain, modified SST and function) that we will judge whether or not this intervention has been successful. So now, we have to create a summary report of your trigger finger. The best way to do this is to complete an additional form but this time, it is an overall impression of your recorded scores.

Tables 3 and 4 summarise the scale and frequency data collected from the diary however, we also need to record function. "Scale data" recorded in table three, relates to the information that is collected from a scale. If we look at the modified SST scale we can see that it is numbered 0 through 5 where a rising score indicates a poor quality of movement. The PNRS is a scale that has zero at one end and 10 on the other thereby creating an 11-point scale where by zero is the lowest score and 10 is the highest score meaning that the higher the score, the greater the perceived pain. These are therefore called scale measurements.

"Frequency data" all those data that need to be counted each time they occur. They cannot be classed as a scale as they do not appear on a discreet, named measurement however, we can say that the more frequently the problem occurs, the worse the problem generally is. However, using a frequency measure does not necessarily tell you how intense the problem is as being woken at night as in the case of disturbed sleep, if you were awake for three hours this would be worse than being awake for 10 minutes however this level of intensity is not captured because each of these occurrences would be counted as one disturbance. So, although recording these data are useful, they are not without their problems unless they are further refined but to do so, given that we are looking at broad outcome measures, this does not really matter. This is because at the end of the day, we want all of these scales, whether they be scale or frequency, to head towards zero.

Table 4: Summary of Scaled Objective Markers

Week \ Metric	Start/End of week	Movement Quality			Pain					
		SST			PNRS					
		W▲	A♦	P■	WR+	WA▲	AR⊡	AA♦	PR✖	PA■
Week 0 Baseline	Day 1[a]									
	Day 7									
Week 1 Resting Splint	Day 1									
	Day 7									
Week 2 Water Immersion	Day 1									
	Day 7									
Week 3 Tendon Gliding (1)*	Day 1									
	Day 7									
Week 3 Tendon Gliding (2)*	Day 1									
	Day 7									
Week 3 Tendon Gliding (3)*	Day 1									
	Day 7									
Week 4 Forearm Massage 1	Day 1									
	Day 7									
+4-days Forearm Massage 2	Day 1									
	Day 7									
+4-days Forearm Massage 3	Day 1									
	Day 7									
+4-days Forearm Massage 4	Day 1									
	Day 7[b]									
Final Assessment	Day 1[a]									
	Day 7[b]									

* This week can repeat depending on outcome of gliding; ▲ on bending and straightening on **waking**; ♦ on bending and straightening during active period; ■ on bending and straightening at pre-sleep period; + at rest on waking; ⊡ at rest during active period; ✖ on rest resting at pre-sleep period.; a First measurement; b Final measurement.

Table 5: Summary of Frequency Objective Markers

Week \ Metric	Start/End of week	Movement Quality			Pain					
		SST			PNRS					
		W▲	A♦	P■	WR+	WA▲	AR⊡	AA♦	PR✖	PA■
Week 0 Baseline	Day 1[a]									
	Day 7									
Week 1 Resting Splint	Day 1									
	Day 7									
Week 2 Water Immersion	Day 1									
	Day 7									
Week 3 Tendon Gliding (1)*	Day 1									
	Day 7									
Week 3 Tendon Gliding (2)*	Day 1									
	Day 7									
Week 3 Tendon Gliding (3)*	Day 1									
	Day 7									
Week 4 Forearm Massage 1	Day 1									
	Day 7									
+4-days Forearm Massage 2	Day 1									
	Day 7									
+4-days Forearm Massage 3	Day 1									
	Day 7									
+4-days Forearm Massage 4	Day 1									
	Day 7[b]									
Final Assessment	Day 1[a]									
	Day 7[b]									

[a] mg = milligrams; * This week can repeat depending on outcome of gliding.

If you would like to see a video of me complete Table 4 and a separate video completing table 5, just follow the links below:

Table 4: https://www.youtube.com/watch?v=trD_xYvzO38

Table 5 https://www.youtube.com/watch?v=ai9l6uO07ec

NOTE: larger versions of Tables 4 and 5 are available in Appendix 4.

The summary scores in Tables 4 are essentially those that you recorded at the start and end of the seven-day cycle (day 1 and day 7) for each of the weeks presented on a single form. Although I have made a suggestion of how this might look, (see Table 4) as a suggested format you can make up your own and you can even, for those who are inclined, enter this data directly onto a spreadsheet to create charts. I will not go into how to do this as that would be beyond the scope of this book. The recording of data for Table 5 data is slightly different as the data are recorded at the start of the week only for all data points including the final measure at 12 weeks. While we have a frequency measure of this, it is very superficial as scores go as it does not provide us with any detail about the functional problems that may be encountered as a result of trigger finger and so we need to provide subjective accounts which are generally more difficult to record.

However, you may remember that I asked you to write down an activity or function that you found most difficult to do or that you avoided doing. You might say as much or as little about this as you wished as a subjective narrative but now is the time to decide whether or not this function has changed and how it has changed. To that extent, what we are doing is assessing whether the scores that have been recorded over the previous weeks match, or reflect, our functional capabilities. Surprisingly, it could be possible to see changes in the SST and PNRS scores but no change in function. This is mainly due to the objective changes not being of sufficient magnitude however, with large changes in these scores, this nearly always correlate with improved function. Given that a correlation with the more objective metrics isn't always achieved, I want you to decide on the success or otherwise of your functional problem in the following way. Look at the following statements that are numbered below. Read these and decide which one best reflects the situation with regard to your chosen functional activity.

My functional problems is:

0. Worse now compared to how it was at the start of this process.
1. Just the same as it was at the start of this process.
2. Probably slightly better than it was at the start of this process.
3. Certainly better than it was at the start of this process.
4. Much better than it was at the start of this process.
5. Almost back to normal.
6. Back to normal.

The only problem with this scale, is that if you did not have any functional problems prior to starting this process, but only had mild objective problems, in the form of quality of movement and pain, then this functional measure is not appropriate and therefore you do not need to do it to decide on whether or not your trigger finger has improved. You should only use the objective measures of the PNRS and the SST scales.

However, the big question is, what happens if this has not worked. If there has been no change on the SST score or the PNRS score or this concocted functional scale. What if things have got worse? Well, to be honest, this condition tends to get worse with time anyway so for some, just standing still is tantamount to an improvement! However, we will not count it as such. So, in the event that any of these has occurred, what should you do next? The first obvious answer to this is that you continue along established guidelines for the treatment of trigger finger which amount to injections and surgery. However, bearing in mind that you are reading this book, it is assumed that you have either already had one or the other and it has failed, or that you didn't welcome the prospect of either and had sought a more naturalistic approach. If you are still disinclined to have an injection or surgery, there is another alternative which is the ManTTr® Protocol[5]. This is a new form of treatment for trigger finger which is designed to be used by health professionals and body workers to treat trigger finger. I devised the ManTTr® Protocol in 2022 after I acquired trigger finger. The full story of my journey is documented in my book "Manual Therapy Trigger Finger (ManTTr®) Protocol: The natural way to treat trigger finger"[5].

Although it requires a third party to deliver this protocol, I was of the view, when writing the book, that most people either know, or know of, somebody who is a bodyworker of some kind whether that be a physiotherapist, osteopath, chiropractor, masseur, structural integrationist, or other kind of bodyworker that might be interested in undertaking this relatively simple, clearly documented approach. Of course, there are contraindications and precautions related to this sort of intervention as it is quite forceful and so it is very important that whoever should do this, is suitably qualified. In my book on the ManTTr® Protocol, I give clear instructions about who this can be performed on and who it must not be done on and I also offer a brand-new theoretical underpinning for trigger finger and I clearly describe the mechanism by which the ManTTr® Protocol purports to operate thereby providing clinicians, undertaking this on their patients or clients, with a sound theoretical basis thereby underpinning their clinical reasoning for the interventions utilised within the ManTTr® Protocol.

The approach contains only physical interventions and does not require any kinds of pills or potions or medications or injections or surgery. From that standpoint, ManTTr® Protocol is completely naturalistic. It also allows people who undertake it, should it fail, to continue along standard treatments in the field, namely steroid injections and surgery, so at the end of the day, there is nothing to lose by finding out more about the ManTTr® Protocol!

So now we have come to the end of the beginning of this journey. I hope for many of you this series of self-help interventions has been successful and if not, I hope that there are things that you can take away from this book which will help you in the future. However, even in the event that you have improved or not improved to the extent that you would have hoped, you might want to consider this only the end of the beginning of the journey and that should you have the chance to undertake the ManTTr® Protocol, presuming that you do not have any contraindications to its application, this will be another means by which you can make progress.

Finally, I would be truly delighted to hear from anybody who has any comments about this book or perhaps even has any questions about trigger finger or even if you would like to share your trigger finger story with me and your experience of various treatments you have tried, including the treatments in this book. If you would like to contact me, then please do so via the e-mail which is given at the end of this book. Please put "trigger finger self-help" in the subjects line. I'm sure you realise that I receive a lot of messages and correspond only with those people who use the appropriate subject headings. That way, it keeps the SPAM to a minimum!

Thank you for buying and reading this book and I hope to hear from you should you wish to contact me.

References

1. Amirfeyz R, McNinch R, Watts A, Glassey N, Bullock J, Rodriigues J, Davis T. Evidence based management of adult trigger digits. *British Society for Surgery of the Hand Evidence for Surgical Treatment (BEST)*: BSST; 2016.
2. Wright S, Heathcote K, Wright G, Yellen M, Shu-Kay N. Fear of needles. *Australian Journal for General Practitioners.* 2009;38:172-176.
3. Greenfeld P. NHS wields the axe on 17 'unnecessary procedures'. *Guardian*. On-Line: Guardian Media Group; 2018.
4. Mooney HP. Cut useless medical treatments, says Audit Commission. *BMJ : British Medical Journal.* 2011;342.
5. Davidson I. *Manual Therapy Trigger Finger (ManTTr®) Protocol. The natural way to treat trigger finger.* Stockport UK: Physioseye; 2023.
6. Peters-Veluthamaningal C, van der Windt DAWM, Winters JC, Meyboom- de Jong B. Corticosteroid injection for trigger finger in adults. *Cochrane Database of Systematic Reviews.* 2009.
7. Fiorini HJ, Tamaoki MJ, Lenza M, Gomes dos Santos JB, Faloppa F, Belloti JC. Surgery for trigger finger. *Cochrane Database of Systematic Reviews.* 2018.
8. Lunsford D, Valdes K, Hengy S. Conservative management of trigger finger: A systematic review. *J Hand Ther.* 2019;32:212-221.
9. Makkouk AH, Oetgen ME, Swigart CR, Dodds SD. Trigger finger: etiology, evaluation, and treatment. *Current Reviews in Musculoskeletal Medicine.* 2008;1:92-96.
10. Quinnell RC. Conservative management of trigger finger. *Practitioner.* 1980;224:187-190.
11. Patel MR, Bassini L. Trigger fingers and thumb: When to splint, inject, or operate. *The Journal of Hand Surgery.* 1992;17:110-113.
12. Diep D, Chen KJQ, Kumbhare D. Ultrasound-guided interventional procedures for myofascial trigger points: a systematic review. *Reg Anesth Pain Med.* 2021;46:73-80.
13. Ajimsha MS, Shenoy PD, Gampawar N. Role of fascial connectivity in musculoskeletal dysfunctions: A narrative review. *J Bodyw Mov Ther.* 2020;24:423-431.
14. Mann CJ, Perdiguero E, Kharraz Y, Aguilar S, Pessina P, Serrano AL, Muñoz-Cánoves P. Aberrant repair and fibrosis development in skeletal muscle. *Skelet Muscle.* 2011;1:21.
15. Akhtar S, Bradley MJ, Quinton DN, Burke FD. Management and referral for trigger finger/thumb. *BMJ.* 2005;331:30-33.
16. NHS. Treatment Trigger Finger2022.
17. White S, McCullough MBA, Akangah PM. The Structural Effects of Diabetes on Soft Tissues: A Systematic Review. 2021;49:11-27.
18. Wyatt LH, Ferrance RJ. The musculoskeletal effects of diabetes mellitus. *J Can Chiropr Assoc.* 2006;50:43-50.
19. Radu A-F, Bungau SG. Management of Rheumatoid Arthritis: An Overview. *Cells.* 2021;10:1-33.
20. Roddy E, Choi HK. Epidemiology of gout. *Rheum Dis Clin North Am.* 2014;40:155-175.
21. Kumar N, Zhang NJ, Cherepanov D, Romanus D, Hughes M, Faller DV. Global epidemiology of amyloid light-chain amyloidosis. *Orphanet Journal of Rare Diseases.* 2022;17:278.
22. Hara Y, Tajiri Y, Kawano K, Hoshikawa S, Kita Y. The Tenosynovitis of Fingers Associated with Transthyretin Amyloidosis. *The Journal of Hand Surgery (Asian-Pacific Volume).* 2020;25:340-344.

23. Terruzzi I. Muscle Tissue in Hypothyroidism and Hyperthyroidism. In: Luzi L, ed. *Thyroid, Obesity and Metabolism: Exploring Links Between Thyroid Function, Obesity, Metabolism and Lifestyle*. Cham: Springer International Publishing; 2021:209-219.

24. Gyawali P, Takanche JS, Shrestha RK, Bhattarai P, Khanal K, Risal P, Koju R. Pattern of thyroid dysfunction in patients with metabolic syndrome and its relationship with components of metabolic syndrome. *Diabetes Metab J.* 2015;39:66-73.

25. Khatiwada S, Kumar Sah S, KC R, Baral N, Lamsal M. Thyroid dysfunction in metabolic syndrome patients and its relationship with components of metabolic syndrome. *Clin Diabetes Endocrinol.* 2016;2:1-5.

26. NICE. Carpal Tunnel Syndrome. Vol 2023: The National Institute for Health and Care Excellence; 2022:Clinical Knowledge Summaries.

27. Lee SK, Bae KW, Choy WS. The relationship of trigger finger and flexor tendon volar migration after carpal tunnel release. *Journal of Hand Surgery (European Volume).* 2014;39:694-698.

28. NICE. Dupuytren's Disease. *Clinical Knowledge Summaries.* Vol 2023: National Institute for Health and Care Excellence; 2022.

29. Ramchandani J, Thakker A, Tharmaraja T. Time to Reconsider Occupation Induced De Quervain's Tenosynovitis: An Updated Review of Risk Factors. *Orthop Rev (Pavia).* 2022;14:1-6.

30. Hassan K, Sohn A, Shi L, Lee M, Wolf JM. De Quervain Tenosynovitis: An Evaluation of the Epidemiology and Utility of Multiple Injections Using a National Database. *The Journal of Hand Surgery.* 2022;47:284.e281-284.e286.

31. Celik B, Tomatsu SC, Tomatsu S, Khan SA. Epidemiology of mucopolysaccharidoses update. *Diagnostics.* 2021;11:273.

32. Fisher RC, Horner RL, Wood VE. The hand in mucopolysaccharide disorders. *Clinical Orthopaedics and Related Research®.* 1974;104:191-199.

33. Langer D, Maeir A, Michailevich M, Luria S. Evaluating Hand Function in Clients with Trigger Finger. *Occup Ther Int.* 2017;2017:1-8.

34. Davidson I, Crooks K, Newington L, Pilling M, Todd C. Assessing the feasibility of mobilisation of C0–C3 cervical segments to reduce headache in migraineurs. *International Journal of Therapy and Rehabilitation.* 2018;25:382-394.

35. Watson DH, Drummond PD. Head pain referral during examination of the neck in migraine and tension-type headache. *Headache: The Journal of Head and Face Pain.* 2012;52:1226-1235.

36. Watson DH, Drummond PD. Cervical referral of head pain in migraineurs: effects on the nociceptive blink reflex. *Headache: The Journal of Head and Face Pain.* 2014;54:1035-1045.

37. Ragoowansi R, Acornley A, Khoo CT. The Percutaneous trigger finger release: the 'lift-cut' technique. *British Journal of Plastic Surgery.* 2005;58:817-821.

38. Onder G, Pellicciotti F, Gambassi G, Bernabei R. NSAID-related psychiatric adverse events: who is at risk? *Drugs.* 2004;64:2619-2627.

39. Leow MQ, Zheng Q, Shi L, Tay SC, Chan ESY. Non-steroidal anti-inflammatory drugs (NSAIDs) for trigger finger. *Cochrane Database of Systematic Reviews.* 2021.

40. Sytsma TT, Greenlund LK, Greenlund LS. Joint Corticosteroid Injection Associated With Increased Influenza Risk. *Mayo Clinic Proceedings: Innovations, Quality & Outcomes.* 2018;2:194-198.

41. Bindu S, Mazumder S, Bandyopadhyay U. Non-steroidal anti-inflammatory drugs (NSAIDs) and organ damage: A current perspective. *Biochemical Pharmacology.* 2020;180:114147.

42. Fowler C. Do nonsteroidal anti-inflammatory drugs impair tissue healing? *Jaapa.* 2018;31:1-5.

43. Lisowska B, Kosson D, Domaracka K. Positives and negatives of nonsteroidal anti-inflammatory drugs in bone healing: the effects of these drugs on bone repair. *Drug Des Devel Ther.* 2018;12:1809-1814.
44. Wongrakpanich S, Wongrakpanich A, Melhado K, Rangaswami J. A Comprehensive Review of Non-Steroidal Anti-Inflammatory Drug Use in The Elderly. *Aging Dis.* 2018;9:143-150.
45. Ussai S, Miceli L, Pisa FE, Bednarova R, Giordano A, Della Rocca G, Petelin R. Impact of potential inappropriate NSAIDs use in chronic pain. *Drug Des Devel Ther.* 2015;9:2073-2077.
46. Bernard BP, Putz-Anderson V. *Musculoskeletal disorders and workplace factors; a critical review of epidemiologic evidence for work-related musculoskeletal disorders of the neck, upper extremity, and low back.* Cincinnati: National Institute for Occupational Safety and Health Publications Dissemination; 1997.
47. Finniss D, Nicholas M, Brooker C, Cousins M, Benedetti F. Magnitude, response, and psychological determinants of placebo effects in chronic low-back pain: a randomised, double-blinded, controlled trial. *Pain Rep.* 2019;4:e744.
48. Diener HC, Dodick DW, Aurora SK, Turkel CC, DeGryse RE, Lipton RB, Silberstein SD, Brin MF. OnabotulinumtoxinA for treatment of chronic migraine: Results from the double-blind, randomized, placebo-controlled phase of the PREEMPT 2 trial. *Cephalalgia.* 2010;30:804-814.
49. Aurora SK, Dodick DW, Turkel CC, DeGryse RE, Silberstein SD, Lipton RB, Diener HC, Brin MF. OnabotulinumtoxinA for treatment of chronic migraine: Results from the double-blind, randomized, placebo-controlled phase of the PREEMPT 1 trial. *Cephalalgia.* 2010;30:793-803.
50. Armstrong TJ, Chaffin DB. Some biomechanical aspects of the carpal tunnel. *Journal of Biomechanics.* 1979;12:567-570.
51. Diller RB, Tabor AJ. The Role of the Extracellular Matrix (ECM) in Wound Healing: A Review. *Biomimetics (Basel).* 2022;7:1-15.
52. Avery JC, Richards LG. Comparison of Trigger Finger Orthotic Wearing Schedules: A Feasibility Study. *Physical & Occupational Therapy In Geriatrics.* 2021;39:182-205.
53. Nakano J, Yamabayashi C, Scott A, Reid WD. The effect of heat applied with stretch to increase range of motion: a systematic review. *Phys Ther Sport.* 2012;13:180-188.

APPENDIX 1: Constructing and Applying a 'DIY' Splint

The following photographs are a step-by-step guide on how to make a trigger finger splint from very basic materials. The materials that are required are: an old piece of cloth (in this case a piece of cotton material) a pair of scissors, a rigid board (in this case, a wooden lolly stick) and tape (in this case, paper based medical tape). These are shown in photo A1.

Photos A1 i-xxxv: Making your own finger splint

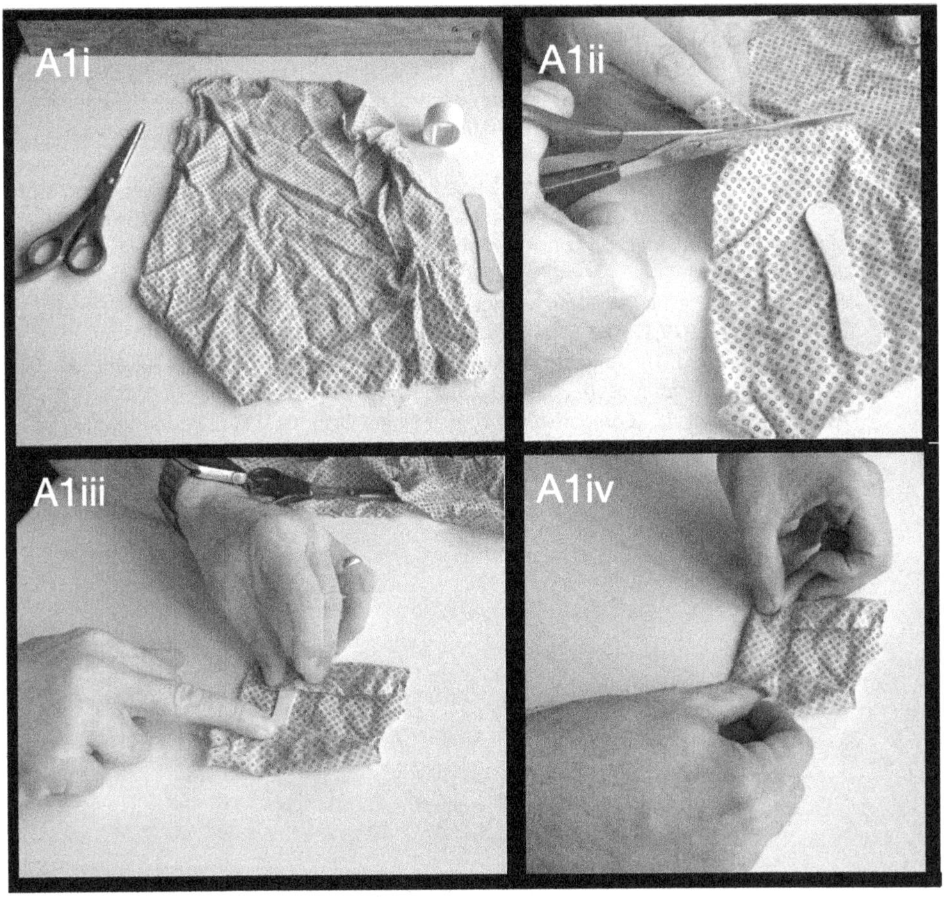

Place the rigid board on the cloth and cut out a generous piece making sure that the cloth can be overlapped over the board (A1ii). Then fold the cloth over both ends of the rigid board (A1iii) and then fold the cloth up until the rigid board has been completely enveloped by the cloth (A1iv-vi). Anchor the ends of the cloth covered rigid bar at both ends using the paper medical tape (A1vii—x) and tear off the tape (A1xi).

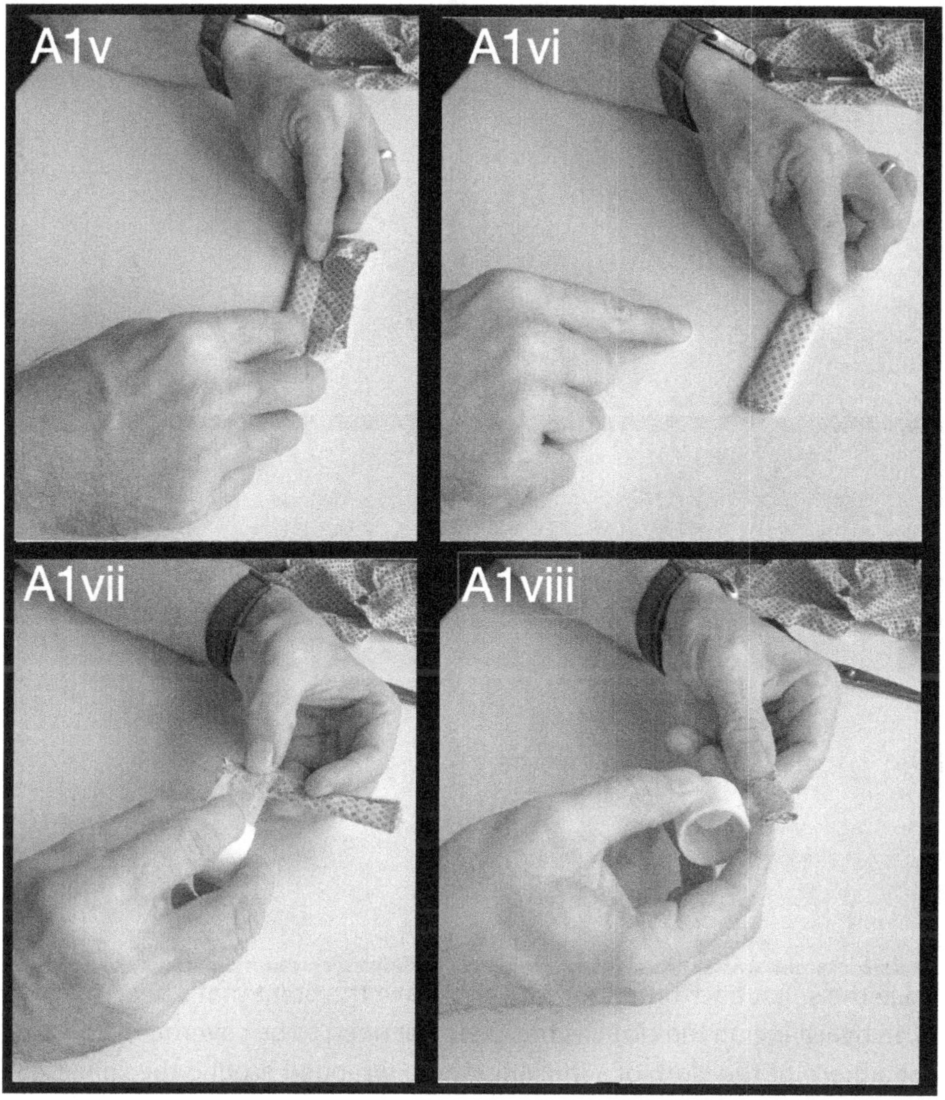

The splint should now look like photo A1xii. Place this over the affected finger and measure a point on the splint over the first joint of the finger (A1xiii-xiv).

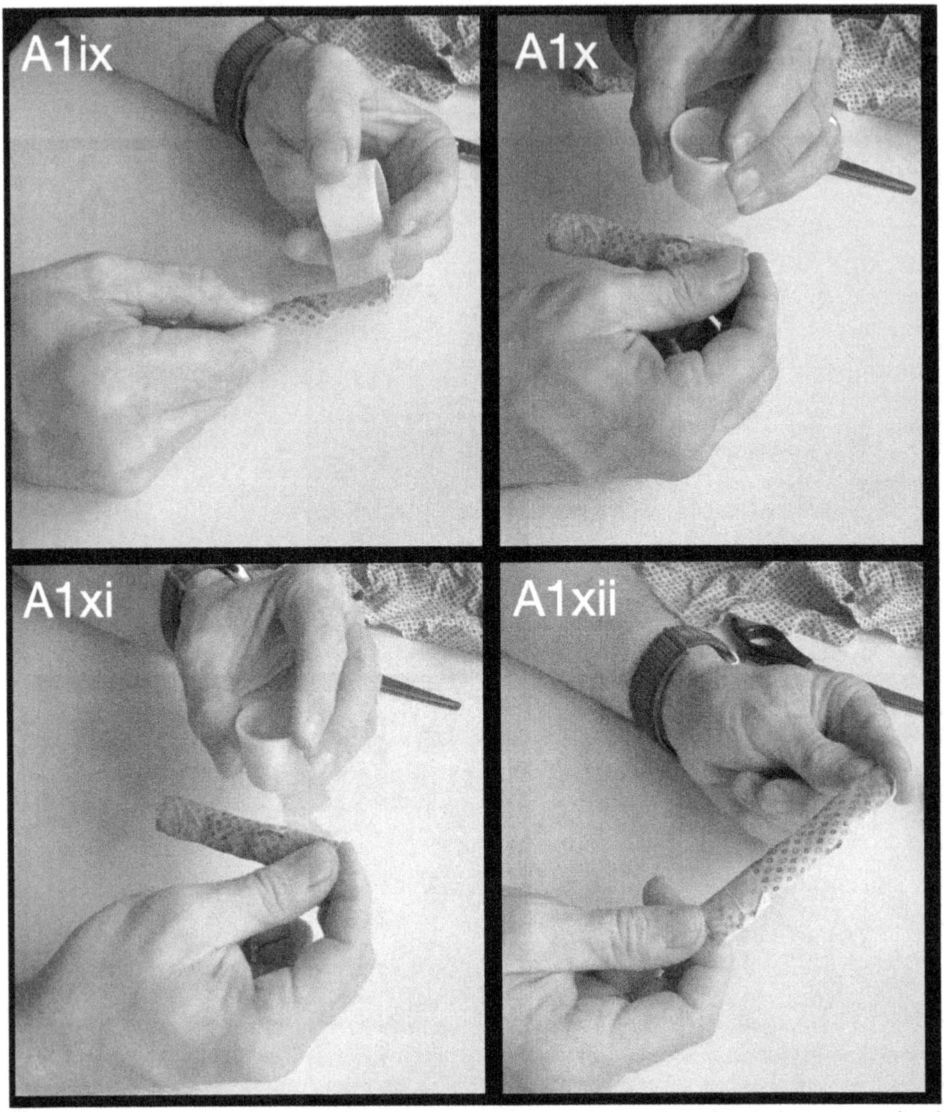

Place the splint back onto the cloth and leave the point that's been marked as an overhang on the cloth as this does not need to be covered (A1xv). Cut out a piece of the cloth of sufficient size to wrapped around the splint and the finger (A1xvi-xviii)

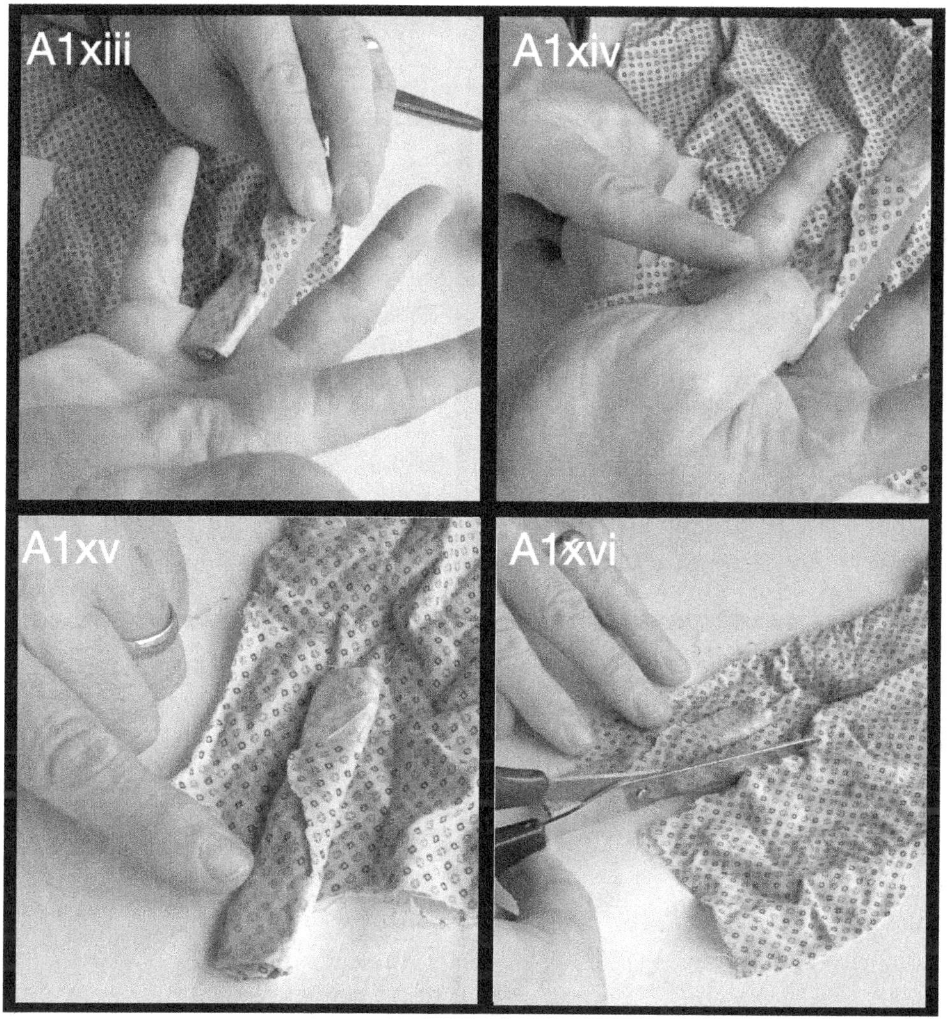

Make sure that the folded end on the stick is uppermost (A1xix-xx) and attach one side of the recently cut out piece of cloth along the middle of the splint using the medical tape (A1xxi- A1xxiv). Put the splint and the attached cloth on the tabletop (A1xxv) and place the affected finger on the splint (A1xxvi).

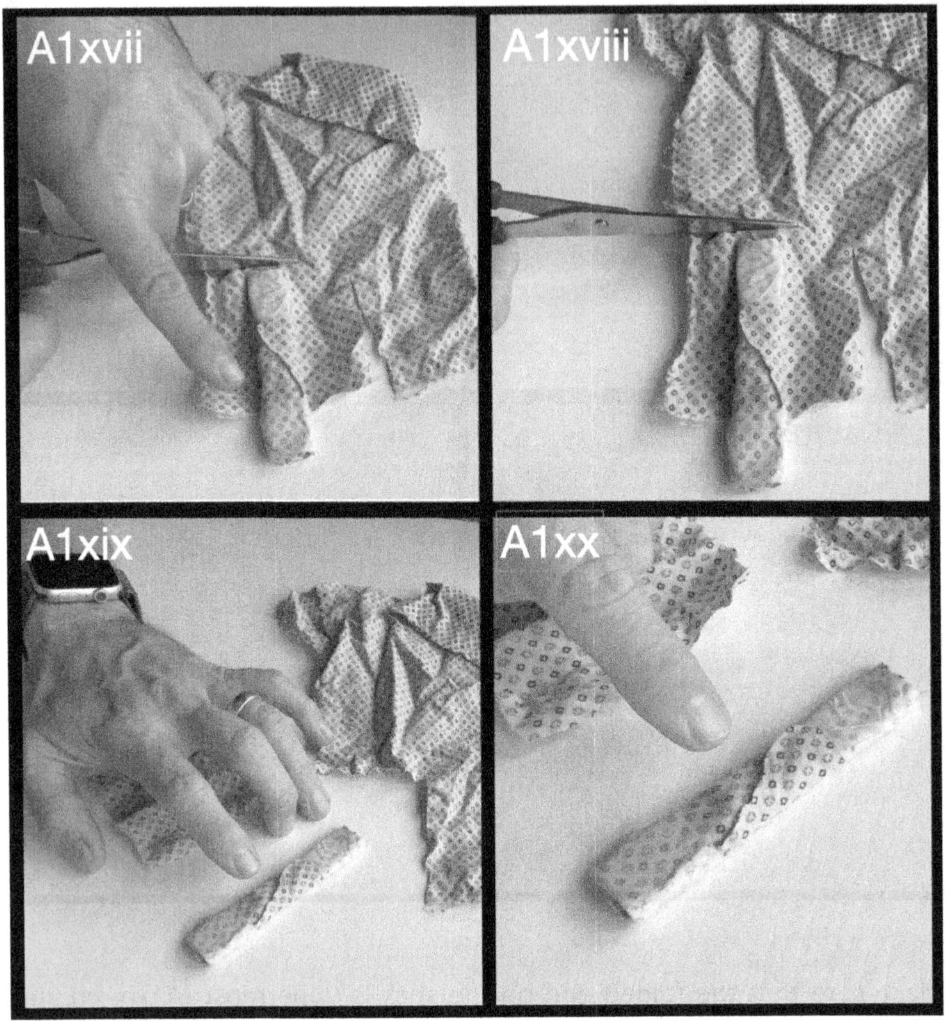
A1xvii
A1xviii
A1xix
A1xx

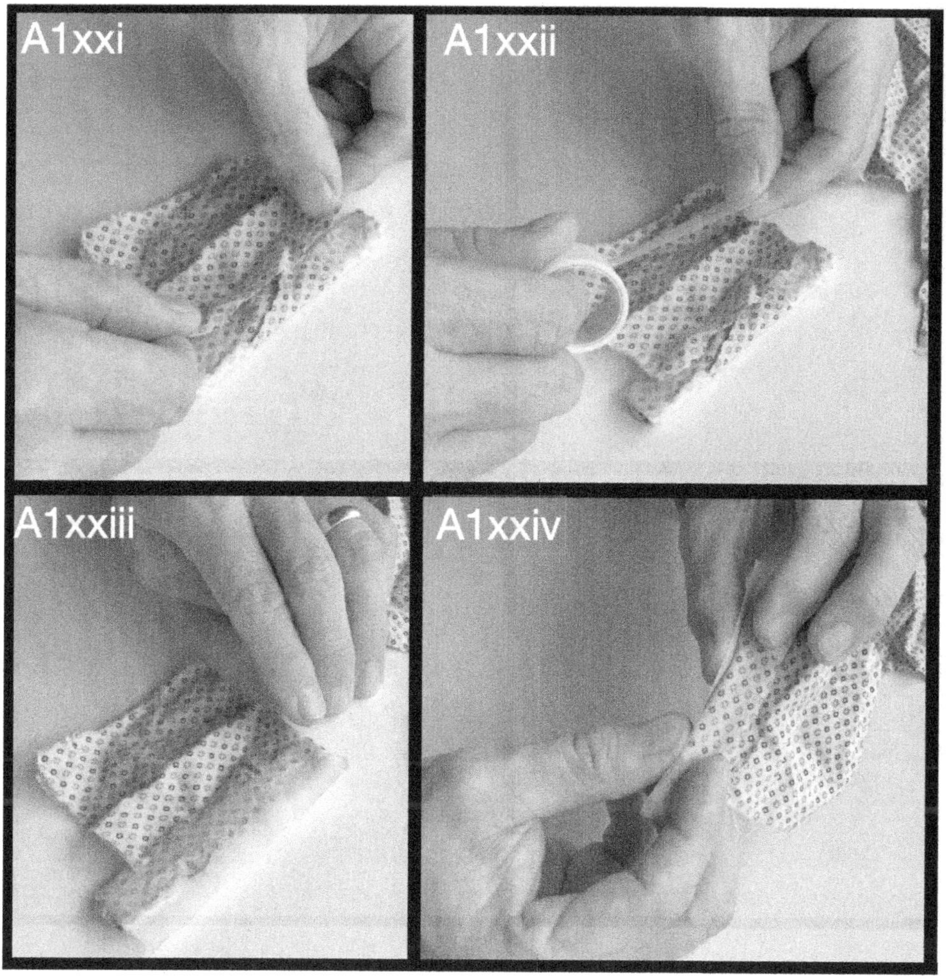
A1xxi
A1xxii
A1xxiii
A1xxiv

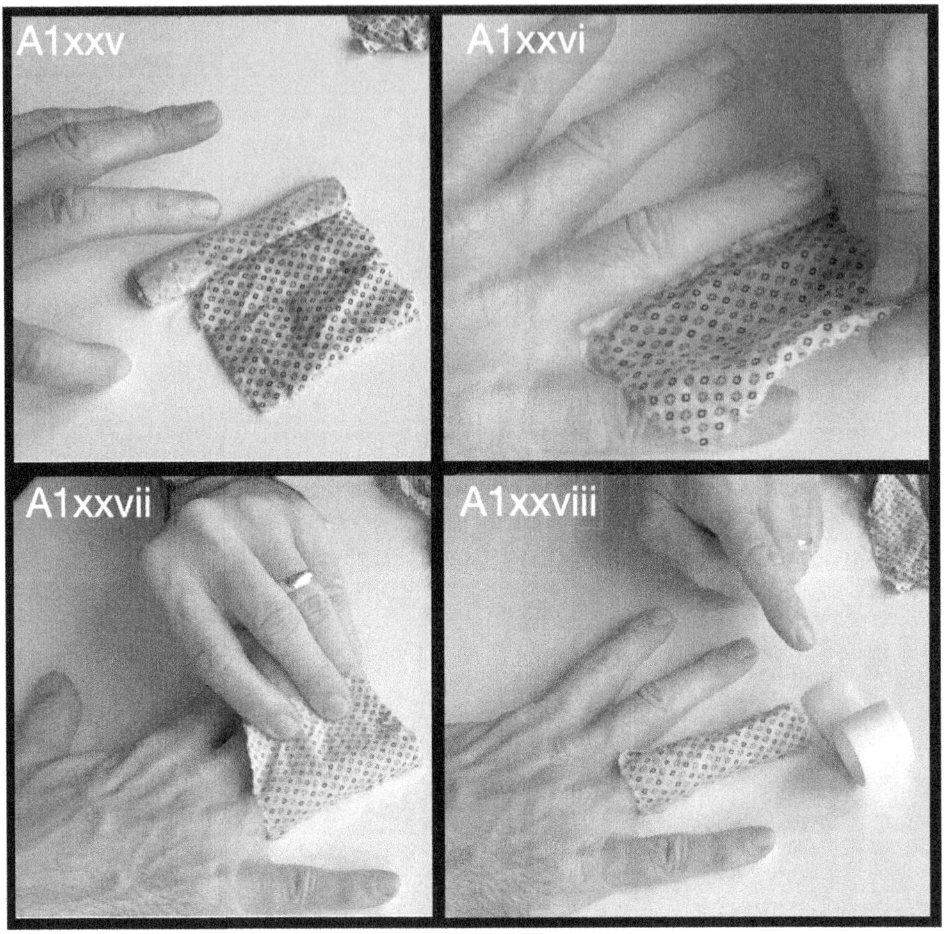

Wrap the excess cloth around the finger and tuck underneath the back of the splint and hold in that position by applying downward pressure through the finger (A1xxvii).

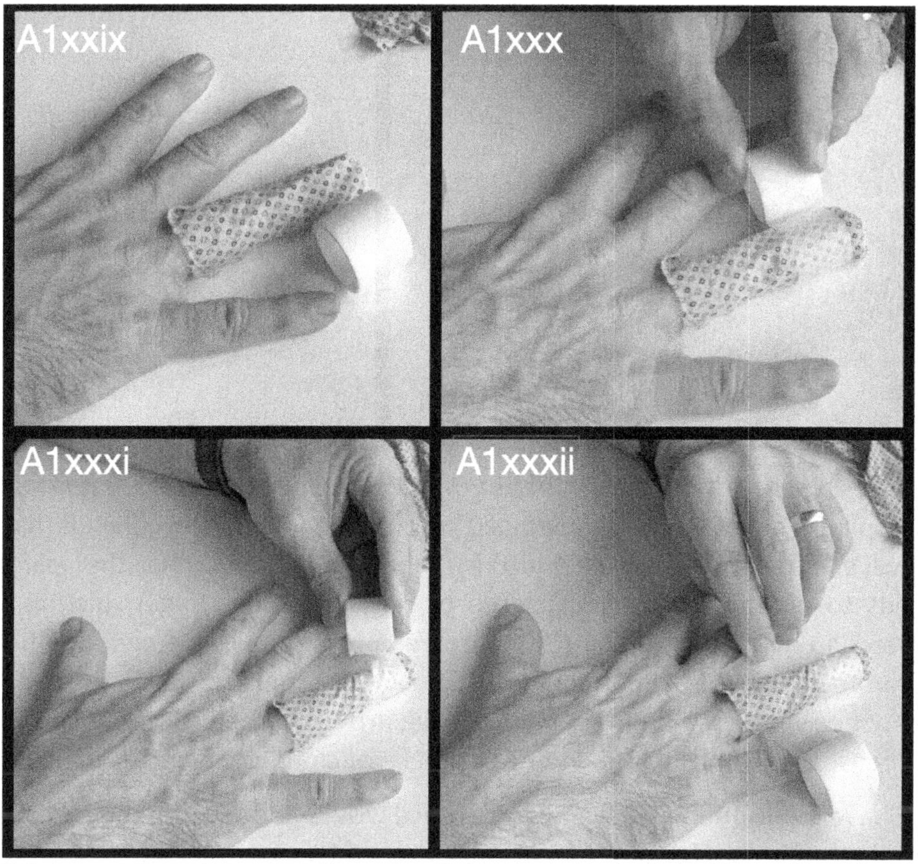

Prior to doing that, unroll some of the tape and place it on the tabletop with the sticky side facing upwards (A1xxviii). Then place the wrapped finger over the tape and wind around 1 full revolution with moderate tension and anchor the end part of the finger (A1xxix-A1xxxii). Finally, tie off the other end of the splint and check for comfort (A1xxxiii-xxxv).

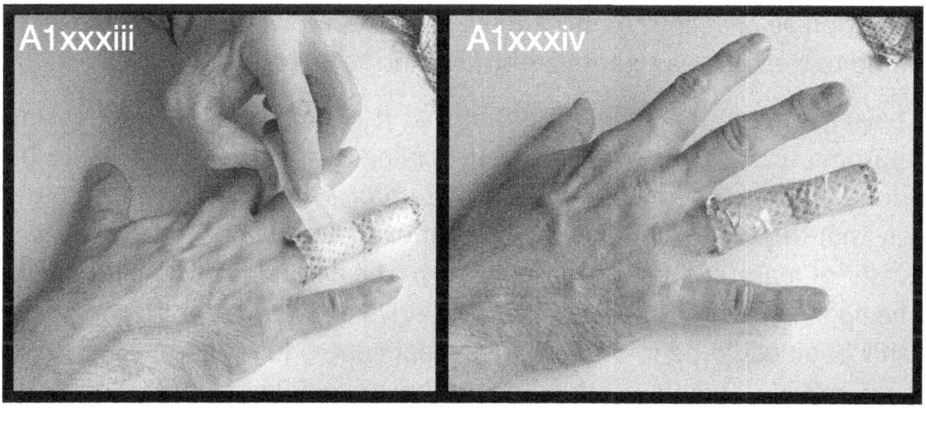

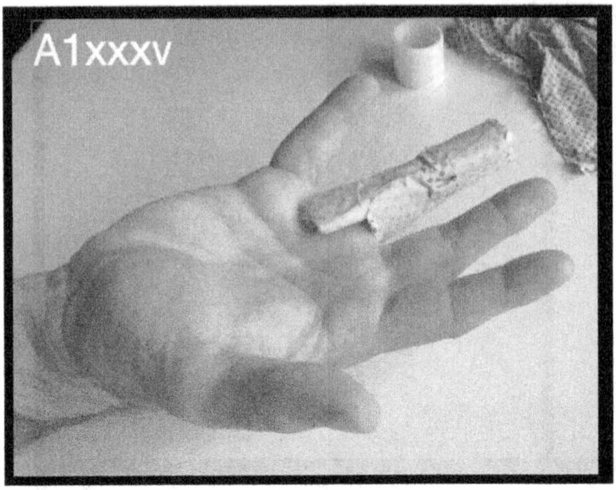

As you can see, there are a number of stages involved in the creation of this splint. Some of you might think that this is an overly complex design however, there is reason behind this. The main reason is that the splint needs to provide not just a degree of rigidity for the finger, but also protection of the skin. As in this case, we're using tape, this needs to be separated from the skin as some people can develop a rash as a result of the adhesive even though, in this case we are using medical tape. This is the reason why I have added the extra piece of cloth to cover the finger.

As I have mentioned earlier, my preference would be for you to buy an off the shelf splint as this is much easier to don and doff and clean. However, these materials that I have suggested in the construction of the splint are made from things which are likely to be around the house with the exception, possibly, of the medical tape. Other tape can be used however when applying taped to the skin, it is recommended that you use only that which is designed to go against the skin. The extra cloth layer is merely a precaution against any complications. The other downside of using tape is related to the relative tightness of the splint.

If, having applied the splint, you find that it is uncomfortable and giving symptoms such as finger coldness or tingling, then the tape needs to be undone and reapplied. Tape tends to be unforgiving in this regard as it is likely that the tape would need to be removed and reapplied fresh. This is a waste of materials and increases costs particularly since the splint needs to be applied frequently for several weeks. No doubt this design presented in this book could be improved: firstly, applying a foam pad to the splint would provide greater comfort for the finger and, instead of using tape,

Velcro fasteners could be applied. These items are easily available in craft shops however, it can only be bought in minimum quantities which would significantly increase costs. As such, it would only probably be worth making a splint if you already have these materials at hand. However, I feel duty bound to give some indication of how you might make your own splint as I understand that some people have very little money to spend and have to make do with materials that they have readily available. But to reiterate, my recommendation is to buy a finger splint which is "off the shelf" as this is, in the short and medium term, the best course of action.

Finally, on matters of safety, you should ensure that any splint that is worn feels comfortable, and does not produce any additional symptoms. The main symptoms to look for are: coldness in the finger, or pins and needles , skin discolouration or other unfamiliar appearance or sensation in the finger. In fact, if there is anything that you find uncomfortable or unpleasant about wearing the splint, you should remove it. Another potential problem for using a rigid splint is having or making this splint too long. This is potentially dangerous as during the night you might bring your hand up to your face and particularly your eyes and cause damage. As such, the splint should not poke out beyond the tip of the finger and should be fully wound by a protective cloth. Alternatively, a padded finger cover can be used to provide suitable protection. It should be emphasised that the main reason for using a splint is to rest the finger in a straightened position due to the tendency for people with trigger finger to flex into a tight fist during sleep and for this to be evident on waking. The body does this to protect the finger by placing it in what is commonly known as a 'closed posture'. However, this position merely serves to further aggravate and stiffen the finger as it is held in the locked position. Having it rested in the extended, unlocked position, gives it the best chance of settling should there be an inflammatory component present.

It should be noted that although I recommend that you do all of the activities suggested in this book, of all four interventions, the use of a splint is the least important. As an absolute minimum, you could wrap your finger in a finger bandage to the extent that it is difficult to bend the finger into a fist and this may suffice. However, the same precautions apply regarding the safety elements mentioned earlier.

APPENDIX 2: Additional diaries for 'repeat Week 3'

Modified SST (stages of stenosing tenosynovitis) Score Key:
0 Normal finger movement
1 Uneven finger movement (looks smooth but feels rough)
2 Triggering or clicking or catching (looks a bit jerky, not fully smooth)
3 Finger locking in a bent or straight position but can unlock by active finger movements
4 Finger locking in a bent or straight position but unlocked by passive finger movements
5 Locked finger in bent or straightened position but cannot be unlocked at all

Pain Numeric Rating Scale (PNRS) Key:
No pain 0 1 2 3 4 5 6 7 8 9 10 Worst pain Imaginable

Trigger Finger Daily Diary				
Date:		Modified SST score (see Key) 0-5	Pain Level (PNRS) (see key) 0-10	
On waking after main sleep	At rest			
	On bending/straightening			
During most active period	At rest			
	On bending/straightening			
Just prior to main sleep	At rest			
	On bending/straightening			
My trigger finger today has:			Yes	No
	Disturbed my sleep			
	Prevented me from doing an activity I wanted or needed to do			
STATE AND DESCRIBE ACTIVITY:				
Medication for Trigger Finger: Frequency....................times/day **Medication Name: Total daily dose:**			Yes	No
	Can you make a full fist just before my main sleep?			
	Can you straighten your fingers fully just before my main sleep?			

Trigger Finger Daily Diary				
Date:		Modified SST score (see Key) 0-5	Pain Level (PNRS) (see key) 0-10	
On waking after main sleep	At rest			
	On bending/straightening			
During most active period	At rest			
	On bending/straightening			
Just prior to main sleep	At rest			
	On bending/straightening			
My trigger finger today has:			Yes	No
	Disturbed my sleep			
	Prevented me from doing an activity I wanted or needed to do			
STATE AND DESCRIBE ACTIVITY:				
Medication for Trigger Finger: Frequency....................times/day **Medication Name: Total daily dose:**			Yes	No
	Can you make a full fist just before my main sleep?			
	Can you straighten your fingers fully just before my main sleep?			

Trigger Finger Daily Diary			
Date:		Modified SST score (see Key) 0-5	Pain Level (PNRS) (see key) 0-10
On waking after main sleep	At rest		
	On bending/straightening		
During most active period	At rest		
	On bending/straightening		
Just prior to main sleep	At rest		
	On bending/straightening		

My trigger finger today has:	Yes	No
Disturbed my sleep		
Prevented me from doing an activity I wanted or needed to do		
STATE AND DESCRIBE ACTIVITY:		
Medication for Trigger Finger: Frequency...................times/day Medication Name: Total daily dose:	Yes	No
Can you make a full fist just before my main sleep?		
Can you straighten your fingers fully just before my main sleep?		

Trigger Finger Daily Diary			
Date:		Modified SST score (see Key) 0-5	Pain Level (PNRS) (see key) 0-10
On waking after main sleep	At rest		
	On bending/straightening		
During most active period	At rest		
	On bending/straightening		
Just prior to main sleep	At rest		
	On bending/straightening		

My trigger finger today has:	Yes	No
Disturbed my sleep		
Prevented me from doing an activity I wanted or needed to do		
STATE AND DESCRIBE ACTIVITY:		
Medication for Trigger Finger: Frequency...................times/day Medication Name: Total daily dose:	Yes	No
Can you make a full fist just before my main sleep?		
Can you straighten your fingers fully just before my main sleep?		

Trigger Finger Daily Diary			
Date:		Modified SST score (see Key) 0-5	Pain Level (PNRS) (see key) 0-10
On waking after main sleep	At rest		
	On bending/straightening		
During most active period	At rest		
	On bending/straightening		
Just prior to main sleep	At rest		
	On bending/straightening		

My trigger finger today has:	Yes	No
Disturbed my sleep		
Prevented me from doing an activity I wanted or needed to do		
STATE AND DESCRIBE ACTIVITY:		
Medication for Trigger Finger: Frequency....................times/day Medication Name: Total daily dose:	Yes	No
Can you make a full fist just before my main sleep?		
Can you straighten your fingers fully just before my main sleep?		

Trigger Finger Daily Diary			
Date:		Modified SST score (see Key) 0-5	Pain Level (PNRS) (see key) 0-10
On waking after main sleep	At rest		
	On bending/straightening		
During most active period	At rest		
	On bending/straightening		
Just prior to main sleep	At rest		
	On bending/straightening		

My trigger finger today has:	Yes	No
Disturbed my sleep		
Prevented me from doing an activity I wanted or needed to do		
STATE AND DESCRIBE ACTIVITY:		
Medication for Trigger Finger: Frequency....................times/day Medication Name: Total daily dose:	Yes	No
Can you make a full fist just before my main sleep?		
Can you straighten your fingers fully just before my main sleep?		

Trigger Finger Daily Diary				
Date:		Modified SST score (see Key) 0-5	Pain Level (PNRS) (see key) 0-10	
On waking after main sleep	At rest			
	On bending/straightening			
During most active period	At rest			
	On bending/straightening			
Just prior to main sleep	At rest			
	On bending/straightening			
My trigger finger today has:			Yes	No
	Disturbed my sleep			
	Prevented me from doing an activity I wanted or needed to do			
STATE AND DESCRIBE ACTIVITY:				
Medication for Trigger Finger: Frequency....................times/day Medication Name: Total daily dose:			Yes	No
	Can you make a full fist just before my main sleep?			
	Can you straighten your fingers fully just before my main sleep?			

Trigger Finger Daily Diary				
Date:		Modified SST score (see Key) 0-5	Pain Level (PNRS) (see key) 0-10	
On waking after main sleep	At rest			
	On bending/straightening			
During most active period	At rest			
	On bending/straightening			
Just prior to main sleep	At rest			
	On bending/straightening			
My trigger finger today has:			Yes	No
	Disturbed my sleep			
	Prevented me from doing an activity I wanted or needed to do			
STATE AND DESCRIBE ACTIVITY:				
Medication for Trigger Finger: Frequency....................times/day Medication Name: Total daily dose:			Yes	No
	Can you make a full fist just before my main sleep?			
	Can you straighten your fingers fully just before my main sleep?			

Trigger Finger Daily Diary

Date:		Modified SST score (see Key) 0-5	Pain Level (PNRS) (see key) 0-10
On waking after main sleep	At rest		
	On bending/straightening		
During most active period	At rest		
	On bending/straightening		
Just prior to main sleep	At rest		
	On bending/straightening		

My trigger finger today has:	**Yes**	**No**
Disturbed my sleep		
Prevented me from doing an activity I wanted or needed to do		
STATE AND DESCRIBE ACTIVITY:		

Medication for Trigger Finger: Frequency……………….times/day **Medication Name: Total daily dose:**	Yes	No
Can you make a full fist just before my main sleep?		
Can you straighten your fingers fully just before my main sleep?		

Trigger Finger Daily Diary

Date:		Modified SST score (see Key) 0-5	Pain Level (PNRS) (see key) 0-10
On waking after main sleep	At rest		
	On bending/straightening		
During most active period	At rest		
	On bending/straightening		
Just prior to main sleep	At rest		
	On bending/straightening		

My trigger finger today has:	**Yes**	**No**
Disturbed my sleep		
Prevented me from doing an activity I wanted or needed to do		
STATE AND DESCRIBE ACTIVITY:		

Medication for Trigger Finger: Frequency……………….times/day **Medication Name: Total daily dose:**	Yes	No
Can you make a full fist just before my main sleep?		
Can you straighten your fingers fully just before my main sleep?		

Trigger Finger Daily Diary			
Date:		Modified SST score (see Key) 0-5	Pain Level (PNRS) (see key) 0-10
On waking after main sleep	At rest		
	On bending/straightening		
During most active period	At rest		
	On bending/straightening		
Just prior to main sleep	At rest		
	On bending/straightening		

My trigger finger today has:	Yes	No
Disturbed my sleep		
Prevented me from doing an activity I wanted or needed to do		
STATE AND DESCRIBE ACTIVITY:		
Medication for Trigger Finger: Frequency....................times/day Medication Name: Total daily dose:	Yes	No
Can you make a full fist just before my main sleep?		
Can you straighten your fingers fully just before my main sleep?		

Trigger Finger Daily Diary			
Date:		Modified SST score (see Key) 0-5	Pain Level (PNRS) (see key) 0-10
On waking after main sleep	At rest		
	On bending/straightening		
During most active period	At rest		
	On bending/straightening		
Just prior to main sleep	At rest		
	On bending/straightening		

My trigger finger today has:	Yes	No
Disturbed my sleep		
Prevented me from doing an activity I wanted or needed to do		
STATE AND DESCRIBE ACTIVITY:		
Medication for Trigger Finger: Frequency....................times/day Medication Name: Total daily dose:	Yes	No
Can you make a full fist just before my main sleep?		
Can you straighten your fingers fully just before my main sleep?		

Trigger Finger Daily Diary

Date:		Modified SST score (see Key) 0-5	Pain Level (PNRS) (see key) 0-10
On waking after main sleep	At rest		
	On bending/straightening		
During most active period	At rest		
	On bending/straightening		
Just prior to main sleep	At rest		
	On bending/straightening		

My trigger finger today has:	**Yes**	**No**
Disturbed my sleep		
Prevented me from doing an activity I wanted or needed to do		
STATE AND DESCRIBE ACTIVITY:		

Medication for Trigger Finger: Frequency....................times/day **Medication Name: Total daily dose:**	**Yes**	**No**
Can you make a full fist just before my main sleep?		
Can you straighten your fingers fully just before my main sleep?		

Trigger Finger Daily Diary

Date:		Modified SST score (see Key) 0-5	Pain Level (PNRS) (see key) 0-10
On waking after main sleep	At rest		
	On bending/straightening		
During most active period	At rest		
	On bending/straightening		
Just prior to main sleep	At rest		
	On bending/straightening		

My trigger finger today has:	**Yes**	**No**
Disturbed my sleep		
Prevented me from doing an activity I wanted or needed to do		
STATE AND DESCRIBE ACTIVITY:		

Medication for Trigger Finger: Frequency....................times/day **Medication Name: Total daily dose:**	**Yes**	**No**
Can you make a full fist just before my main sleep?		
Can you straighten your fingers fully just before my main sleep?		

APPENDIX 3: Extra Diaries for Massage

Modified SST (stages of stenosing tenosynovitis) Score Key:
0 Normal finger movement
1 Uneven finger movement (looks smooth but feels rough)
2 Triggering or clicking or catching (looks a bit jerky, not fully smooth)
3 Finger locking in a bent or straight position but can unlock by active finger movements
4 Finger locking in a bent or straight position but unlocked by passive finger movements
5 Locked finger in bent or straightened position but cannot be unlocked at all

Pain Numeric Rating Scale (PNRS) Key:

No pain											Worst pain Imaginable
	0	1	2	3	4	5	6	7	8	9	10

Trigger Finger Daily Diary				
Date:		Modified SST score (see Key) 0-5	Pain Level (PNRS) (see key) 0-10	
On waking after main sleep	At rest			
	On bending/straightening			
During most active period	At rest			
	On bending/straightening			
Just prior to main sleep	At rest			
	On bending/straightening			
My trigger finger today has:			Yes	No
	Disturbed my sleep			
	Prevented me from doing an activity I wanted or needed to do			
STATE AND DESCRIBE ACTIVITY:				
Medication for Trigger Finger: Frequency.....................times/day Medication Name: Total daily dose:			Yes	No
	Can you make a full fist just before my main sleep?			
	Can you straighten your fingers fully just before my main sleep?			

Trigger Finger Daily Diary				
Date:		Modified SST score (see Key) 0-5	Pain Level (PNRS) (see key) 0-10	
On waking after main sleep	At rest			
	On bending/straightening			
During most active period	At rest			
	On bending/straightening			
Just prior to main sleep	At rest			
	On bending/straightening			
My trigger finger today has:			Yes	No
	Disturbed my sleep			
	Prevented me from doing an activity I wanted or needed to do			
STATE AND DESCRIBE ACTIVITY:				
Medication for Trigger Finger: Frequency.....................times/day Medication Name: Total daily dose:			Yes	No
	Can you make a full fist just before my main sleep?			
	Can you straighten your fingers fully just before my main sleep?			

Trigger Finger Daily Diary			
Date:		Modified SST score (see Key) 0-5	Pain Level (PNRS) (see key) 0-10
On waking after main sleep	At rest		
	On bending/straightening		
During most active period	At rest		
	On bending/straightening		
Just prior to main sleep	At rest		
	On bending/straightening		

My trigger finger today has:	Yes	No
Disturbed my sleep		
Prevented me from doing an activity I wanted or needed to do		
STATE AND DESCRIBE ACTIVITY:		

Medication for Trigger Finger: Frequency.....................times/day Medication Name: Total daily dose:	Yes	No
Can you make a full fist just before my main sleep?		
Can you straighten your fingers fully just before my main sleep?		

Trigger Finger Daily Diary			
Date:		Modified SST score (see Key) 0-5	Pain Level (PNRS) (see key) 0-10
On waking after main sleep	At rest		
	On bending/straightening		
During most active period	At rest		
	On bending/straightening		
Just prior to main sleep	At rest		
	On bending/straightening		

My trigger finger today has:	Yes	No
Disturbed my sleep		
Prevented me from doing an activity I wanted or needed to do		
STATE AND DESCRIBE ACTIVITY:		

Medication for Trigger Finger: Frequency.....................times/day Medication Name: Total daily dose:	Yes	No
Can you make a full fist just before my main sleep?		
Can you straighten your fingers fully just before my main sleep?		

Trigger Finger Daily Diary			
Date:		Modified SST score (see Key) 0-5	Pain Level (PNRS) (see key) 0-10
On waking after main sleep	At rest		
	On bending/straightening		
During most active period	At rest		
	On bending/straightening		
Just prior to main sleep	At rest		
	On bending/straightening		

My trigger finger today has:	Yes	No
Disturbed my sleep		
Prevented me from doing an activity I wanted or needed to do		
STATE AND DESCRIBE ACTIVITY:		
Medication for Trigger Finger: Frequency...................times/day Medication Name: Total daily dose:	Yes	No
Can you make a full fist just before my main sleep?		
Can you straighten your fingers fully just before my main sleep?		

Trigger Finger Daily Diary			
Date:		Modified SST score (see Key) 0-5	Pain Level (PNRS) (see key) 0-10
On waking after main sleep	At rest		
	On bending/straightening		
During most active period	At rest		
	On bending/straightening		
Just prior to main sleep	At rest		
	On bending/straightening		

My trigger finger today has:	Yes	No
Disturbed my sleep		
Prevented me from doing an activity I wanted or needed to do		
STATE AND DESCRIBE ACTIVITY:		
Medication for Trigger Finger: Frequency...................times/day Medication Name: Total daily dose:	Yes	No
Can you make a full fist just before my main sleep?		
Can you straighten your fingers fully just before my main sleep?		

Trigger Finger Daily Diary			
Date:		Modified SST score (see Key) 0-5	Pain Level (PNRS) (see key) 0-10
On waking after main sleep	At rest		
	On bending/straightening		
During most active period	At rest		
	On bending/straightening		
Just prior to main sleep	At rest		
	On bending/straightening		

My trigger finger today has:	Yes	No
Disturbed my sleep		
Prevented me from doing an activity I wanted or needed to do		
STATE AND DESCRIBE ACTIVITY:		

Medication for Trigger Finger: Frequency....................times/day Medication Name: Total daily dose:	Yes	No
Can you make a full fist just before my main sleep?		
Can you straighten your fingers fully just before my main sleep?		

Trigger Finger Daily Diary			
Date:		Modified SST score (see Key) 0-5	Pain Level (PNRS) (see key) 0-10
On waking after main sleep	At rest		
	On bending/straightening		
During most active period	At rest		
	On bending/straightening		
Just prior to main sleep	At rest		
	On bending/straightening		

My trigger finger today has:	Yes	No
Disturbed my sleep		
Prevented me from doing an activity I wanted or needed to do		
STATE AND DESCRIBE ACTIVITY:		

Medication for Trigger Finger: Frequency....................times/day Medication Name: Total daily dose:	Yes	No
Can you make a full fist just before my main sleep?		
Can you straighten your fingers fully just before my main sleep?		

Trigger Finger Daily Diary			
Date:		Modified SST score (see Key) 0-5	Pain Level (PNRS) (see key) 0-10
On waking after main sleep	At rest		
	On bending/straightening		
During most active period	At rest		
	On bending/straightening		
Just prior to main sleep	At rest		
	On bending/straightening		

My trigger finger today has:	Yes	No
Disturbed my sleep		
Prevented me from doing an activity I wanted or needed to do		
STATE AND DESCRIBE ACTIVITY:		
Medication for Trigger Finger: Frequency.....................times/day **Medication Name: Total daily dose:**	Yes	No
Can you make a full fist just before my main sleep?		
Can you straighten your fingers fully just before my main sleep?		

Trigger Finger Daily Diary			
Date:		Modified SST score (see Key) 0-5	Pain Level (PNRS) (see key) 0-10
On waking after main sleep	At rest		
	On bending/straightening		
During most active period	At rest		
	On bending/straightening		
Just prior to main sleep	At rest		
	On bending/straightening		

My trigger finger today has:	Yes	No
Disturbed my sleep		
Prevented me from doing an activity I wanted or needed to do		
STATE AND DESCRIBE ACTIVITY:		
Medication for Trigger Finger: Frequency.....................times/day **Medication Name: Total daily dose:**	Yes	No
Can you make a full fist just before my main sleep?		
Can you straighten your fingers fully just before my main sleep?		

Trigger Finger Daily Diary			
Date:		Modified SST score (see Key) 0-5	Pain Level (PNRS) (see key) 0-10
On waking after main sleep	At rest		
	On bending/straightening		
During most active period	At rest		
	On bending/straightening		
Just prior to main sleep	At rest		
	On bending/straightening		

My trigger finger today has:	Yes	No
Disturbed my sleep		
Prevented me from doing an activity I wanted or needed to do		
STATE AND DESCRIBE ACTIVITY:		
Medication for Trigger Finger: Frequency..................times/day **Medication Name: Total daily dose:**	Yes	No
Can you make a full fist just before my main sleep?		
Can you straighten your fingers fully just before my main sleep?		

Trigger Finger Daily Diary			
Date:		Modified SST score (see Key) 0-5	Pain Level (PNRS) (see key) 0-10
On waking after main sleep	At rest		
	On bending/straightening		
During most active period	At rest		
	On bending/straightening		
Just prior to main sleep	At rest		
	On bending/straightening		

My trigger finger today has:	Yes	No
Disturbed my sleep		
Prevented me from doing an activity I wanted or needed to do		
STATE AND DESCRIBE ACTIVITY:		
Medication for Trigger Finger: Frequency..................times/day **Medication Name: Total daily dose:**	Yes	No
Can you make a full fist just before my main sleep?		
Can you straighten your fingers fully just before my main sleep?		

Trigger Finger Daily Diary

Date:		Modified SST score (see Key) 0-5	Pain Level (PNRS) (see key) 0-10
On waking after main sleep	At rest		
	On bending/straightening		
During most active period	At rest		
	On bending/straightening		
Just prior to main sleep	At rest		
	On bending/straightening		

My trigger finger today has:	Yes	No
Disturbed my sleep		
Prevented me from doing an activity I wanted or needed to do		
STATE AND DESCRIBE ACTIVITY:		

Medication for Trigger Finger: Frequency....................times/day Medication Name: Total daily dose:	Yes	No
Can you make a full fist just before my main sleep?		
Can you straighten your fingers fully just before my main sleep?		

Trigger Finger Daily Diary

Date:		Modified SST score (see Key) 0-5	Pain Level (PNRS) (see key) 0-10
On waking after main sleep	At rest		
	On bending/straightening		
During most active period	At rest		
	On bending/straightening		
Just prior to main sleep	At rest		
	On bending/straightening		

My trigger finger today has:	Yes	No
Disturbed my sleep		
Prevented me from doing an activity I wanted or needed to do		
STATE AND DESCRIBE ACTIVITY:		

Medication for Trigger Finger: Frequency....................times/day Medication Name: Total daily dose:	Yes	No
Can you make a full fist just before my main sleep?		
Can you straighten your fingers fully just before my main sleep?		

Trigger Finger Daily Diary				
Date:		Modified SST score (see Key) 0-5	Pain Level (PNRS) (see key) 0-10	
On waking after main sleep	At rest			
	On bending/straightening			
During most active period	At rest			
	On bending/straightening			
Just prior to main sleep	At rest			
	On bending/straightening			

My trigger finger today has:	Yes	No
Disturbed my sleep		
Prevented me from doing an activity I wanted or needed to do		
STATE AND DESCRIBE ACTIVITY:		
Medication for Trigger Finger: Frequency...................times/day Medication Name: Total daily dose:	Yes	No
Can you make a full fist just before my main sleep?		
Can you straighten your fingers fully just before my main sleep?		

Trigger Finger Daily Diary				
Date:		Modified SST score (see Key) 0-5	Pain Level (PNRS) (see key) 0-10	
On waking after main sleep	At rest			
	On bending/straightening			
During most active period	At rest			
	On bending/straightening			
Just prior to main sleep	At rest			
	On bending/straightening			

My trigger finger today has:	Yes	No
Disturbed my sleep		
Prevented me from doing an activity I wanted or needed to do		
STATE AND DESCRIBE ACTIVITY:		
Medication for Trigger Finger: Frequency...................times/day Medication Name: Total daily dose:	Yes	No
Can you make a full fist just before my main sleep?		
Can you straighten your fingers fully just before my main sleep?		

APPENDIX 4: Tables 4 and 5 Enlarged

Table 3

Metric / Week	Start/End of week	Movement Quality			Pain					
		SST			PNRS					
		W▲	A♦	P■	WR+	WA▲	AR⊡	AA♦	PR✖	PA■
Week 0 Baseline	Day 1[a]									
	Day 7									
Week 1 Resting Splint	Day 1									
	Day 7									
Week 2 Water Immersion	Day 1									
	Day 7									
Week 3 Tendon Gliding (1)*	Day 1									
	Day 7									
Week 3 Tendon Gliding (2)*	Day 1									
	Day 7									
Week 3 Tendon Gliding (3)*	Day 1									
	Day 7									
Week 4 Forearm Massage 1	Day 1									
	Day 7									
+4-days Forearm Massage 2	Day 1									
	Day 7									
+4-days Forearm Massage 3	Day 1									
	Day 7									
+4-days Forearm Massage 4	Day 1									
	Day 7[b]									
Final Assessment	Day 1[a]									
	Day 7[b]									

* This week can repeat depending on outcome of gliding; ▲ on bending and straightening on **waking**; ♦ on bending and straightening during active period; ■ on bending and straightening at pre-sleep period; + at rest on waking; ⊡ at rest during active period; ✖ on rest resting at pre-sleep period.; a First measurement; b Final measurement.

Table 4

Week \ Metric	Start/End of week	Movement Quality: SST W▲	A♦	P■	Pain: PNRS WR+	WA▲	AR⊡	AA♦	PR✖	PA■
Week 0 Baseline	Day 1[a]									
	Day 7									
Week 1 Resting Splint	Day 1									
	Day 7									
Week 2 Water Immersion	Day 1									
	Day 7									
Week 3 Tendon Gliding (1)*	Day 1									
	Day 7									
Week 3 Tendon Gliding (2)*	Day 1									
	Day 7									
Week 3 Tendon Gliding (3)*	Day 1									
	Day 7									
Week 4 Forearm Massage 1	Day 1									
	Day 7									
+4-days Forearm Massage 2	Day 1									
	Day 7									
+4-days Forearm Massage 3	Day 1									
	Day 7									
+4-days Forearm Massage 4	Day 1									
	Day 7[b]									
Final Assessment	Day 1[a]									
	Day 7[b]									

[a] mg = milligrams; * This week can repeat depending on outcome of gliding.

About the Author

Ian Davidson was born in Wallasey on the Wirral Peninsular. He has been a physiotherapist in the UK for 40 years as a clinician, teacher, researcher and practice owner. He lives in Stockport, Greater Manchester, UK with his wife and family.

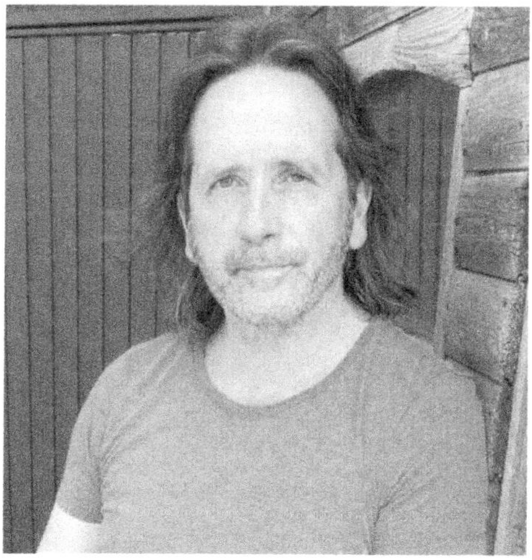

Other titles by this author:

Manual Therapy Trigger Finger (ManTTr®) Protocol: The natural way to treat trigger finger

Contact the Author at: neuro.msk.physio@gmail.com

Made in the USA
Monee, IL
04 November 2026

67383104R10085